COMPLIANCE
The Dilemma of the Chronically Ill

Kenneth E. Gerber, Ph.D., is Director of the Pain Management Program at the Long Beach Veterans Administration Medical Center, Long Beach, California. He is a member of the clinical faculty at the University of California at Los Angeles as well as an Instructor in the Psychology Department at California State University, Long Beach. He has research and teaching interests in the areas of gerontology, hemodialysis, and pain control.

Alexis M. Nehemkis, Ph.D., also a member of the psychology staff of the Veterans Administration Medical Center, Long Beach, California, is a member of the clinical faculty of the Department of Psychology at the University of Southern California. She was formerly affiliated with the Los Angeles Suicide Prevention Center and has served as a behavioral consultant to the Los Angeles County Medical Examiner-Coroner's office. She is the author of numerous articles on the psychological correlates, prediction and measurement of chronic pain and cancer pain, self-destructive patterns in chronic illness, and medical staff attitudes and bias.

Compliance
The Dilemma of the Chronically Ill

Kenneth E. Gerber, Ph.D.
Alexis M. Nehemkis, Ph.D.

EDITORS

SPRINGER PUBLISHING COMPANY
New York

Springer Publishing Company, Inc.
536 Broadway
New York, New York 10012

86 87 88 89 90 / 5 4 3 2 1

Library of Congress Cataloging-in-Publication Data
Main entry under title:

Compliance : the dilemma of the chronically ill.

  Includes bibliographies and index.
  1. Patient compliance. 2. Chronic diseases—
Psychological aspects. I. Gerber, Kenneth E.
II. Nehemkis, Alexis M. [DNLM: 1. Chronic
Diseases—psychology. 2. Patient Compliance.
W 85 C7375]
R726.5.C645 1986   616   85-26041
ISBN 0-8261-4580-9

Printed in the United States of America

To my parents, Daniel and P.G.

K.E.G.

To Barbara and Viva

A.M.N.

Contents

Contributors   ix

Foreword by Atara Kaplan De-Nour   xi

Acknowledgments   xv

1 **Prologue: The Dilemma of the Chronically Ill**   3
   Kenneth E. Gerber and Alexis M. Nehemkis

2 **Compliance in the Chronically Ill: An
   Introduction to the Problem**   12
   Kenneth E. Gerber

3 **Noncompliance as Indirect Self-Destructive
   Behavior**   24
   Norman L. Farberow

4 **Adherence: A Cognitive-Behavioral
   Perspective**   44
   Dennis C. Turk, Peter Salovey, and Mark D. Litt

5 **Compliance and the Quality of Survival**   73
   Alexis M. Nehemkis and Kenneth E. Gerber

   Family Relationships and Compliance   98
   Amy Herstein Gervasio

7   The Special Case of Compliance in the
    Elderly   128
        Phyllis L. Amaral

8   The Eye of the Beholder: Staff Perceptions of
    Noncompliance   158
        Alexis M. Nehemkis

9   Physician-Patient Communication and
    Compliance   182
        Richard W. Hanson

10 How Society Contributes to Noncompliance   213
        Carol Cummings and Alexis M. Nehemkis

11 Epilogue: The Complex Nature of
    Compliance   226
        Kenneth E. Gerber and Alexis M. Nehemkis

Index   236

Contributors

Phyllis L. Amaral received her Ph.D. in clinical-aging psychology. She currently serves as Director of Research and Evaluation at The Center for the Partially Sighted in Santa Monica, California.

Carol Cummings received her Ph.D. from the University of California, Los Angeles, in 1975. Formerly Director of Psychological Services at the Centinela Hospital Pain Management Center in Inglewood, California, she is currently affiliated with the New Hope Pain Center in Pasadena, California. Dr. Cummings has lectured widely on the psychological aspects of chronic pain and has published articles on the psychological assessment and treatment of chronic pain.

Norman L. Farberow's career as a clinical/research psychologist has focused on the problem of suicide and its prevention. As co-founder and co-director of the Los Angeles Suicide Prevention Center and as Clinical Professor of Psychiatry (Psychology) at the University of Southern California School of Medicine, he has helped develop clinical services; trained professionals, paraprofessionals, and nonprofessionals; and conducted research into all aspects of suicide for over 30 years. He has been President of the International Association for Suicide Prevention and the American Association of Suicidology as well as relevant divisions in the American Psychological Association and other psychology associations. He has co-authored and edited 160 publications in the field of suicide, including 13 books.

Amy Herstein Gervasio, who received her Ph.D. in clinical psychology from Ohio State University, is currently Assistant Professor of Psychology at Hamilton College in Clinton, New York. Her clinical interests include the psychological effects of illness on spinal-cord injured, kidney, stroke, and oncology patients. She has conducted research on the linguistic properties of behavior therapy and on everyday memory in neurologically impaired patients.

Richard W. Hanson, Ph.D., is Assistant Chief and Director of the Psychology Training Program at the Veterans Administration Medical Center, Long Beach, California. He is also Clinical Assistant Professor at the University of California at Los Angeles and Clinical Associate Professor at the University of Southern California. Dr. Hanson's current teaching, research, and clinical interests are in the area of behavioral medicine with special emphasis on the management of stress and chronic pain.

Mark D. Litt, M.A., is a doctoral candidate in clinical psychology at Yale University and is a Psychology Associate at the West Haven Veterans Administration Medical Center Pain Management Program. His current research areas include occupational stress and worker health, cognitive-behavioral interventions in pain and illness, and behavioral pediatrics.

Peter Salovey, M.A., is a doctoral candidate in clinical psychology at Yale University where he conducts research in the areas of health cognition and the effects of mood states on behavior. He recently completed a book with V. J. D'Andrea entitled *Peer Counseling: Skills and Perspectives.*

Dennis C. Turk, Ph.D., is Associate Professor of Psychology at Yale University, where he has been a faculty member since 1977. He is also Director of the Pain Management Laboratory and Research Clinic at Yale and a consultant to the Pain Management Program at the West Haven Veterans Administration Medical Center. Dr. Turk has published widely in the area of behavioral medicine and recently published a book with D. H. Meichenbaum and M. Genest entitled *Pain and Behavioral Medicine: A Cognitive-Behavioral Perspective.*

Foreword

Hundreds of articles and dozens of books have been written about patients' compliance, and most of them are reviewed or mentioned in this book. Yet the need for more information and for better understanding is great because the management of this problem is still poor, and 50 percent of patients are still noncompliers.

Compliance: The Dilemma of the Chronically Ill has highlighted some of the crucial problems: Compliance has many facets, and most patients are not either good or bad compliers but may comply or adhere perfectly to one aspect of the medical–rehabilitation regimen while drastically abusing another one. As long as we regard all patients' behavior as either compliant or noncompliant, little progress will be made. I was made aware of this many years ago when I was in charge of our outpatient department of psychiatry. This was (and still is) a multidisciplinary—and because of our population—a multilingual service. At the time when Mrs. A. B. came for screening, our French-speaking professional was absent. Being in charge, I interviewed her myself, in school French, easily diagnosed a major affective disorder, decided to put her on amitriptyline, and explained to her the plan of treatment. During the following few weeks Mrs. A. B. came to see me regularly, received the prescriptions with the explanation for gradual increase in medication, etc., and greatly improved. Four months later the treatment was terminated with great success, and still a year later she was invited for a check-up. During the brief interview she expressed her gratitude at her recovery. Just before leaving she removed from her handbag a big plastic bag with *all* the amitriptyline—she had not taken a single pill! I was so annoyed that I asked her why on earth she had come so regularly, to which she answered, "Your French, doctor, was so funny that it made me feel good." I did not ask her in French why she had not taken the medication.

This rather silly story is just an addition to what has been elaborated on in the book—that patients may comply with parts of the regimen and that we should aim at obtaining information about their differential compliance with the various aspects of the treatment program.

The book highlights a second and even more important issue: Noncompliance should be regarded as a nonspecific symptom, like fever, and the factors that cause or contribute to noncompliance are numerous. The patient's background, personality, conscious or unconscious forces, the family of the patient, the treating physician, and the medical team are only a few of the factors that may promote compliance or noncompliance. There is some evidence about the influence of most factors, though the information occasionally is contradictory. However, comprehensive studies focusing simultaneously on a number of factors suggested to influence compliance are lacking. It is hoped that this book, with its presentation of the many factors of noncompliance, will motivate such comprehensive studies.

Linked to this problem is the third important issue: If we indeed accept that noncompliance is determined by many factors, we cannot expect to improve compliance by any one method of intervention. Actually, any and every noncompliant patient should be diagnosed as to the etiology of noncompliance in his or her specific case. Only then can rational interventions be suggested, tailored according to the patient's problem and not to our orthodox orientation, be it dynamic psychotherapy, behavior modification, changing staff attitudes, or social policy.

I would like to add that I believe *Compliance: The Dilemma of the Chronically Ill* may unintentionally highlight the problem which, to me, is the most important one: Not a single M.D. participated in the writing of this book. Most of the very interesting studies reported here were published in psychological and social journals, few in psychiatric journals, and still fewer in medical, nonpsychiatric journals. We the physicians are treating an aging population of patients with mostly chronic diseases. We prescribe and recommend and, in our different styles, communicate with the patients and tell them what to do. But are we aware of the fact that we hardly have a 50 percent chance of the patients complying with our suggestions, recommendations, and orders? One might suggest that the only shortcoming of the book is its title. Perhaps it should have been called *Compliance: The Dilemma of the Medical Profession.*

ATARA KAPLAN DE-NOUR, M.D.
Chief Psychiatrist
Hadassah Medical Center
Jerusalem, Israel

Acknowledgments

The editors are indebted to many people who have contributed to the ideas of this book as well as to its production. The first editor is especially indebted to Laurina Hildering, with whom he worked during the initial months of this project. She significantly contributed to the book's early development. The editors also gratefully acknowledge the encouragement received from their Chief, Louis Mutalipassi. Appreciation is also due to Barbara Watkins, our editor at Springer, for her assistance. Finally, the editors are especially grateful to Virginia Largent, who conscientiously typed portions of the manuscript. Although we are greatly sympathetic to the ultimate objective of altering conventional English in the nonsexist direction, we have used the generic pronoun "he" to avoid the awkward double pronoun construction or the use of "they" as a singular pronoun.

KEG
AMN

COMPLIANCE
The Dilemma of the Chronically Ill

1

Prologue: The Dilemma of the Chronically Ill

Kenneth E. Gerber
Alexis M. Nehemkis

The dilemma of the chronically ill arises when the demands of long-term illness conflict with the values and needs that patients have developed during their lifetimes. The tensions inherent in this dilemma are often seen in the relations between patients and medical staff and frequently revolve around the issue of compliance. Patients are, in actuality, often noncompliant in their behavior. This behavior, as Dr. Kaplan De-Nour notes in her Foreword, is multidetermined and, for the most part, poorly understood.

Each noncompliant patient's unique situation must be examined without resorting to categorization within only one underlying theoretical orientation. Rather, the clinician must appreciate the myriad of interpersonal, familial, cultural, and situational factors which affect each individual. Only when such influences are understood can appropriate clinical interventions be designed and prescribed.

This book has evolved from the experiences of the editors as clinical psychologists working with medical patients within a large general hospital. As psychological consultants to a variety of medical specialty units, we have often been concerned with assessing and treating the noncompliant chronically ill patient. We have worked extensively with end-stage renal disease patients, oncology patients, nursing home elderly, and chronic pain patients. Our behavioral training has provided us with a framework for the use of rigorous methods of behavioral assessment and treatment with patient groups. However, this perspective has often provided less than satisfactory answers for an understanding of the psychological parameters of compliance in these patient populations. A multidimensional approach to dealing with the issue of compliance in the chronically ill must be considered.

A brief example of the issues faced in the area of hemodialysis will help orient the reader. The hemodialysis unit presents daily reminders of the dramatic and pervasive impact of chronic illness. We have found that many of the responsibilities of psychologists in the dialysis unit center around the issue of compliance. The first contacts with patients involve education about renal disease and dialysis treatment. These sessions are designed to ensure patients' understanding of the seriousness of their condition and of appropriate behavior (e.g., diet restrictions, the importance of not missing dialysis treatments, etc.). Psychological assessments, including family interviews, are conducted to help predict patient compliance once dialysis begins. Treatment interventions are designed to resolve emotional and behavioral obstacles to patient acceptance of dialysis as an inevitable life change. Behavioral indicators of psychological adjustment to dialysis are constantly monitored. Core symptoms of noncompliance, such as eating forbidden foods, being late for treatment, and overindulging in fluids, are noted and targeted for intervention.

It is clear, however, that the issue of compliance rests not only with the patient but also with the interaction of others with this individual. In particular, the role of the staff is critical. Staff expectations of patient behavior are frequently unrealistically high or presented in a confusing manner (Alexander, 1975). Staff judgment of patients as noncompliant is often based on a narrowly defined set of behavioral criteria complicated by an assortment of personal staff preferences for certain types of patients (i.e., more friendly patients can be more noncompliant to diet before actually being labelled as such, in comparison with less outgoing individuals — see Chapter 8 for a description of a research study based on these clinical observations). Staff frequently become depressed, frustrated, and angry when patients are seen as being noncompliant. Staff work earnestly to save the lives of their patients and yet see these efforts seemingly made more difficult by the patients themselves.

However, staff often forget the severe emotional, social, and psychological consequences of dialysis and the strain that this places on the patient. Expectations must be tempered by the reality of the situation, which encompasses the myriad of factors and influences that must be considered by the clinician. It is clear that the degree of patient compliance is the result of a complex interaction of staff expectations, family response, patient age, rigors of the treatment regimen, physician communication skills, and the subjective experiences (i.e., values, beliefs about the quality of daily life, etc.) of the patient as treatment progresses.

As our notion of noncompliance evolved into that of a complex, multidetermined phenomenon, the behavioral interventions we had used to resolve this problem in our chronically ill patients appeared to us to be more and more limited. The clinical strategies we used were efficacious for certain patients whose values and future time orientation were similar to that of educated professional staff. These patients almost always appeared to be compliant but, if not, could benefit from simple informational or educational interventions. Many other patients, however, shared a different perspective on the self-denial and future emphasis orientation that was necessary for them to accept their medical regimen. Such noncompliers were immediately viewed as having psychological problems. These psychological problems, however, were often the result of differences between staff expectations and patient goals.

The issue of compliance is clearly a multidimensional one, with a complex set of factors that affect the behavior of the chronically ill patient. The topics selected in this volume represent those influences that we see as critical in patient compliance. The broadened perspective that these chapters provide will enable the reader to more fully understand and appreciate the area of patient compliance. The topics to be covered are briefly addressed in the following sections.

NONCOMPLIANCE AS INDIRECT SELF-DESTRUCTIVE BEHAVIOR

Farberow, in Chapter 3, discusses the way in which the concept of indirect self-destructive behavior allows us a particular theoretical framework within which to examine noncompliance. Menninger (1938) originally used the term "partial suicide," which has evolved into the term "indirect self-destructive behavior." This concept describes the phenomena of risk taking, poor frustration tolerance, and a predominantly present orientation which is found in the noncompliant patient (Farberow et al., 1970). Delineation of the processes characterizing the seemingly self-destructive act of noncompliance to medical regimens may give the clinician a better grasp of the patient's underlying values and attitudes which determine such behavior. Farberow integrates research results with a theoretical explanation of noncompliant behavior, and produces a portrait of the intraindividual dynamics of noncompliance. His conclusions reinforce the view of such behavior as complex, multidetermined, and, at times, self-affirming.

THE COGNITIVE-BEHAVIORAL APPROACH

The cognitive-behavioral approach recognizes the critical role of implicit beliefs, values, expectations, and self-concept in determining behavior. Meichenbaum (1982) uses the term "current concerns" to illustrate the importance of the patient's phenomenological experience in influencing compliance. These current concerns are seen as critical factors which, if ignored, will ensure the failure of the intervention. Within this framework one finds an emphasis on the importance of being sensitive to such factors. The further concern for self-responsibility and individual choice are enlightened additions to behavioral philosophy. Turk, Salovey, and Litt, in Chapter 4, address the need for an intervention-focused approach which incorporates, rather than ignores, the multiple influences affecting compliant behavior.

QUALITY OF LIFE

Any examination of compliance in chronic illness must consider the subjective experience of the patient. Although such an observation may appear trite, one often hears health care personnel comment that they could not understand why patients had difficulty giving up certain foods, or stopping smoking, if this would allow them to live a longer life. Intensive efforts are needed to help staff appreciate the enormous difficulty patients have in giving up significant aspects of their lives in order to live a longer life which they perceive as highly unrewarding. Many patients cannot find suitable replacements for satisfying aspects of lifelong, often culturally determined lifestyles.

Our work with dialysis and cancer patients has demonstrated the need for examining the phenomenological world of the patient. It is helpful to consider Yalom's (1980) use of May's phrase "disciplined naiveté" — the attempt to understand the private world of the patient without judging this world from a host of our own prejudices. The experience of hemodialysis intensifies those individual concerns classically associated with existentialism: isolation, impending death, responsibility, and the need for meaning. That these issues could be ignored by clinicians in their work with patients suffering from chronic yet terminal diseases seems naive and unacceptable. Such topics are neither untouchable nor anathema to a broad-spectrum cognitive-behavioral clinical approach. Receptivity to such areas enhances the psychologist in the eyes of the patient, if only by contrast with the unwillingness of the medical profession to speak of these issues. Awareness of a patient's private world and appreciation of the individual's values and preferences are certain to facilitate later clinical intervention. There is also the need to help medical staff accept the patient who decides to be noncompliant to some degree as a conscious, self-affirmative choice (Zaner, 1980). Chapter 5 addresses clearly the issues involved in compliance and quality of life and the critical nature of this area for the health care professional.

COMPLIANCE AND THE FAMILY

Litman (1974) has argued that the family is the basic unit of health care. Chronic illness clearly has a pervasive impact on the entire family. It is reasonable to assume that the family can facilitate or obstruct the chronic patient's adaptation to his illness. Although there has recently been a significant growth of interest in family systems theory (Minuchin, 1980), this work generally has not been systematically applied to the family with a chronically ill member. Furthermore, the field of behavioral medicine also has not fully recognized the family as a critical force behind patient coping behavior. For example, a recent review of the behavioral medicine perspective on adherence does not consider the impact of the family (Epstein & Cluss, 1982).

The dearth of work in this area is one of the most significant shortcomings of the chronic illness research literature. Examples of family influences on patient compliance are plentiful in the day-to-day experience of the health professional: the diabetic's wife who believes it her responsibility to police her husband's diet; the dialysis patient's wife who must seek employment for the first time after her husband becomes too ill to work; and the dialysis patient's children who refuse to believe the seriousness of their father's illness and criticize him for being overly concerned about his eventual need for dialysis. Gervasio, in Chapter 6, outlines theoretical views on family interaction in general and, in particular, focuses on clinical manifestations of the family's impact on coping with chronic illness. Her perspective will go a long way towards filling the gap in this area in the literature.

THE ELDERLY CHRONICALLY ILL

The elderly suffer disproportionately from the effects of chronic illness. This population also presents a special health care challenge, in that it is increasing as an overall percentage of the total population. In the Veterans Administration system, for example, World War II veterans are now reaching the age of 65 and are appearing in medical centers with a complex array of chronic physical complaints which the staff has not previously had to handle on a large scale.

In addition to these trends, there are the unique medical, social, and psychological complications of aging, such as dementia, sensory losses, and decreased financial resources. The elderly are more likely to experience a number of chronic illnesses simultaneously, thereby compounding the stress of accomodating to inevitable physical and cognitive limitations. Technological advances in medicine are clearly adding years to the life-span, but with the likelihood of patients continuing to live with multiple chronic diseases.

Amaral, in Chapter 7, discusses the unique circumstances that affect coping with chronic illness in the elderly. Failure to understand how aging affects behavior is certain to frustrate the health care professional trying to design a treatment regimen for chronic patients in this age group. With the growth of this segment of the population it is clearly time to examine how the phenomenon of aging influences patient response to long-term medical regimens.

THE PHYSICIAN/STAFF-PATIENT RELATIONSHIP

The work of DiMatteo and DiNicola (1982) has focused attention on the social–psychological processes affecting the physician–patient relationship and compliant behavior. As the primary relationship within the health care system, it is clear that the quality of this interaction greatly influences patients' acceptance of their medical condition. No attempt to understand the compliance of the chronically ill patient can ignore the power of the physician in influencing patient behavior.

It is important to distinguish, however, between the impact of the physician and the effect of other professional staff, particularly nurses (see Chapter 8), on patient compliance. Although the physician, as head of the multidisciplinary team, often lays the foundation for patients' understanding of and attitude toward their illness, other health care staff usually have considerably more contact with patients than the doctor. While the social status and function of the nurse, for example, varies significantly from that of the doctor, the impact of nonphysician health personnel on patient behavior is still clearly very strong.

Recent research has emphasized the importance of the process of staff judgment of patients as noncompliant, when such labeling in part reflects stereotyping and cultural bias. Kaplan De-Nour's (1983) work with dialysis patients succinctly describes the unreasonable expectations, often ambiguously communicated, of nursing staff toward dialysis patients. After years of observing the interaction among patients and staff in dialysis units, Kaplan De-Nour has concluded that noncompliance is a staff problem, reflecting the medical staff's unreasonable expectations of patients facing an incredibly stressful array of social and psychological factors. The impact of staff behavior on a patient being labeled noncompliant is a critical theme throughout this volume (see, in particular, Chapters 5, 8, and 9).

SOCIETAL CONTRIBUTIONS

Health professionals generally work within the relatively narrow confines of the office, outpatient clinic, and hospital. They are, in a sense, somewhat shielded from society as a whole. There are a number of influences that the larger governmental and medical care systems impose upon both health professionals and patients that affect patient compliance. Interestingly, the tangled web of insurance requirements, governmental regulations, and medical constraints often work to reward noncompliance (or, at least, do not reward compliance). For example, patients who adhere to a treatment regimen for low back pain may find themselves becoming functional to the point that they lose eligibility for Social Security benefits, but these individuals will not be hired by many employers due to insurance restrictions. It is important to note Fordyce's (1968) warning of the great obstructive impact of governmental aid programs on patient motivation.

Within the medical care facility, complex and sometimes contradictory treatment regimens, which frequently fail to consider the individual being treated, virtually ensure noncompliance on the part of the patient. On a more general level, the social and cultural influences of medicine, which incorporate often unrealistic expectations of medical intervention on the part of both the patient and the medical professional, contribute to noncompliance. Patients with unrealistically high expectations, perhaps fostered by society at large, will find that their health care includes "failed promises" and will be less motivated to be compliant with treatment regimens in the future. This myriad of societal issues must be dealt with in treating the individual patient and becoming aware of the factors that may potentially influence the degree of compliance of the patient. Cummings and Nehemkis discuss these issues in greater detail in Chapter 10.

REFERENCES

Alexander, L. The double-bind theory and hemodialysis. *Archives of General Psychiatry, 33*, 1353–1356, 1976.

DiMatteo, M., & DiNicola, D. *Achieving patient compliance*. New York: Pergamon, 1982.

Epstein, L., & Cluss, P. A behavioral medicine perspective on adherence to long-term medical regimens. *Journal of Consulting and Clinical Psychology, 50*, 950–971, 1982.

Farberow, N., Darbonne, A., Stein, K., & Hirsch, S. Self-destructive behavior of uncooperative diabetics. *Psychological Reports, 27*, 935–946, 1970.

Fordyce, W., Fowler, Lehmann, L., & DeLateur, B. Some implications of learning in problems of chronic pain. *Journal of Chronic Diseases, 21*, 179–190, 1968.

Kaplan De-Nour, A. Staff-patient interaction. In N. Levy (Ed.), *PsychoNephrology 2*. New York: Plenum, 1983.

Menninger, K. *Man against himself*. New York: Harcourt Brace, 1938.

Minuchin, S. *Families and family therapy*. Cambridge, MA. Harvard University Press, 1974.

Turk, D., Meichenbaum, D., & Genest, M. *Pain and behavioral medicine*. New York: Guilford, 1983.

Witenberg, S., Blanchard, E., McCoy, G., Suls, J., & McGoldrick, M. D. Evaluation of compliance in home and center hemodialysis patients. *Health Psychology, 2*, 227–237, 1983.

Yalom, I. *Existential psychotherapy*. New York: Basic Books, 1980.

Zaner, R. Dialysis and ethics: Be strong and trust (please!). In N. Levy (Ed.), *PsychoNephrology 1*. New York: Plenum, 1981.

2

Compliance in the Chronically Ill: An Introduction to the Problem

Kenneth E. Gerber

Chronic illness is an increasingly significant concern within health psychology (Matarazzo, 1982). The contribution of lifestyle factors to producing much of our chronic disease is now clear, although the most effective remedies for the resolution of these factors remains the subject of much debate. Prevention of chronic disease by alteration of life patterns is receiving strong emphasis through programs examining "risk" factors such as weight and stress. Chronic disease is increasing not only because these risk factors are endemic to many deeply ingrained cultural values, but also because individuals, through medical advances, can now live longer by following certain restrictive regimens. Conditions such as diabetes, renal failure, hypertension, and chronic pain affect millions of individuals (10 million Americans suffer from diabetes, for example), and the task of living with these illnesses can be summarized under the general rubric of "compliance."

COMPLIANCE VS ADHERENCE

Compliance has usually been defined in a general way such as by Haynes (1976): "the extent to which a person's behavior coincides with medical or health advice" (pp. 2-3). The measurement of compliance in clinical settings is, however, controversial. There is often little agreement among health care professionals about what constitutes compliant behavior with any particular medical regimen. The validity and practicality of methods determine whether they will be the chosen measures in any particular clinical setting (Epstein & Cluss, 1982).

Turk et al. in Chapter 4 of this book associates the term compliance with the traditional health care relationship within which the patient is a passive responder to the physician's authoritarian demands. As they view this type of relationship as opposed to the alternative cognitive-behavioral model they propose, they reject compliance in favor of adherence. Adherence denotes a collaborative, interactional relationship. Barofsky (1978) argues that in addition to the terms compliance and adherence can be added a third: "therapeutic alliance." All these terms represent points along a continuum of social control. The medical professional–patient relationship inherently consists of varying degrees of external control of the patient's life by the care provider over the course of treatment. Whereas compliance and adherence usually imply a standard external to both parties, therapeutic alliance implies a negotiated reciprocal agreement between patient and provider which may result from a developing positive social relationship. It is clear, however, that no consensus exists as to which term best describes the behaviors that define a patient's following of medical recommendations. We prefer the more collaborative staff-patient relationship and indeed recognize that the traditional medical model contributes to poor patient compliance (see Hanson, Chapter 9). Throughout this book we continue, however, to use the term compliance by which most health care personnel describe these patient behaviors. Recent research reviews (Epstein & Cluss, 1982; Mazur, 1981) also use the term compliance for the same reason.

THE EXTENT OF NONCOMPLIANCE

Recent extensive literature reviews have delineated the major issues within the general research field of compliance with medical regimen (DiMatteo & DiNicola, 1982; Epstein & Cluss, 1982; Mazur, 1981). Research in the area of compliance includes a wide array of subjects from one individual following the advice of one doctor to take antibiotics for a sore throat to the influence of public health policy on preventive health behaviors (i.e., developing exercise regimen; smoking cessation). In the present work we consider the matter of compliance within one kind of patient population—the chronic physically ill—and many of our case examples are from patients with illnesses such as chronic renal failure, diabetics, cancer, and chronic pain. However, much of the research literature in the general compliance area raises issues relevant to any specific patient group, and a summary of the previous research provides a foundation for the chapters in this work.

It has been well documented that noncompliance is considered a serious health care problem (Becker & Maiman, 1975; Kasl, 1975; Sackett & Haynes, 1976). Sackett (1976) suggests that 50 percent of the patients do not take prescribed medications. Medical appointments are missed from 20 to 50 percent of the time. Recommendations to change habits, including increases in exercise and smoking cessation, for example, show particularly poor compliance rates. Physicians show poor predictive ability in judging whether a patient will be compliant (Haynes, 1976). It is also generally accepted that compliance rates tend to decrease the longer the regimen must be followed. Here we can identify the critical factor of chronicity of condition and its impact on compliance. One study (Bloom, Cerkoney, & Hart, 1980) showed that fewer than 7% of the chronic diabetic patients fully complied with medically recommended self-care procedures. Further research has shown that diabetic patients often follow regimen procedures incorrectly (Watkins, Williams, Martin, Hogan, & Anderson, 1967) as evidenced by misinterpretation of urine test results or self-administering the incorrect dosage of insulin. These research results showing consistently low compliance rates are particularly significant because of the increasing evidence that certain behavior changes can have dramatic impact on the course of chronic disease. In hypertension, for example, proper use of blood pressure medication and adapting an appropriate diet can significantly arrest the damage done by destructive coronary artery disease. Physical complications of unstable, poorly controlled diabetes includes hypo/hyperglycemia, peripheral nerve damage, chronic kidney disease although the exact relationship between noncompliance and physical deterioration is not completely understood. Yet there is considerable evidence that (McKenney, Slining, Henderson, Devins, & Barr, 1973) hypertension medications are often not taken frequently enough or in the correct therapeutic dosage. Research with diabetics confirms that compliance with dietary restriction in this population is also quite poor (Wing, Epstein, & Nowalk, 1984).

FACTORS AFFECTING COMPLIANCE

It is clear that compliance rates vary according to how they are measured. Patient self-report measures have been shown to be significantly inaccurate when compared with objective (e.g., blood tests) tests with the tendency for the more noncomplying patients to be the least accurate in their self-description (Mazur, 1981). More objective measures have shortcomings also. Pill counts, for example, may be affected by patients simply discarding medication rather than their taking appropriate dosage. Biochemical analyses are vulnerable to individual metabolic differences between patients. However, such tests are generally the better of the assessment choices. Medical treatment outcome as a measure of appropriate compliance is clearly affected by diverse and confounding variables (e.g., physical condition at start of treatment) and could not be said to directly assess a patient's compliance level. Since no one measurement method is without inadequacies, caution must be exercised in interpreting research results. In addition, different studies may use differing assessment methods, so comparison of results across studies must be done with care.

Throughout this book authors will be reviewing the myriad of variables identified as influencing compliance with medical regime. Previous literature reviews (Epstein & Cluss, 1982; Mazur, 1981) have concluded that a wide assortment of variables affect compliance rates. Demographic variables have not been consistently shown to relate to compliance. However, with some diseases, higher levels of education and higher social class have been shown to contribute to greater levels of compliance (Tagliacozzo & Ima, 1970). Knowledge of the medical condition does not increase compliance rates, but knowledge of the regimen does (Kirscht & Rosenstock, 1979). More complex medical instructions lowers compliance rates. In addition, compliance rates with one part of the regimen do not predict the patient's adherence to other regimen aspects. Patient–provider relationships appear to be an especially important determinant of compliance (Stone, 1979). Those health professionals who provide consistent care within a caring relationship do seem to influence higher compliance rates in their patients.

Another set of factors affecting compliance could be referred to as individual factors and would consist of the patient's perception of their illness and their sense of control over their condition. Such approaches are cognitive in emphasis and are designed with some modification to include the effects of external variables such as objective health state (Becker, 1974). Other theorists have taken a strict environmentalist view of compliance, viewing adherence to medical regimen as a series of behaviors controlled by externally generated rewards and punishments (Zifferblatt, 1975).

INTERVENTION STRATEGIES TO INCREASE COMPLIANCE

The improvement of compliance rates has been a major treatment concern in the field of health psychology. An assortment of behavioral techniques have been used with limited success. Among these methods are cueing, stimulus control techniques (i.e., flavoring pills to improve taste), self-monitoring methods (i.e., keeping records of pills taken) (Johnson, Taylor, Sackett, Dunnet, & Shinizu, 1978), and reinforcement of medication use and symptom reduction (Haynes, 1976). In reviewing these various behavioral methods, Epstein and Cluss (1982) are critical of the research methods adopted in the studies and conclude that, in general, such techniques do not significantly improve compliance rates.

Other treatment approaches have stressed informational/educational interventions (i.e., meetings with patients to discuss medication, telephone reminders regarding upcoming medical appointments). Such methods have not, generally, improved compliance rates (Kirscht & Rosenstock, 1979). Interventions aimed at improving patient–provider relationships have been identified as holding significant promise for future interventions

(Stone, 1979). Here, improving effective communication skills of medical professionals would be the major treatment focus.

The reviews of compliance literature (Epstein & Cluss, 1982; Kirscht & Rosenstock, 1979; Mazur, 1981; Stone, 1979) generally conclude that compliance rates are the result of complex interactions of many differing factors, many of which have been discussed above. The awareness of this complex multidetermined view of compliance has not always been translated into effective treatment protocols. It seems that attempts to increase compliance have not been impressive as a consequence of failing to consider the multiplicity of factors affecting compliance.

Even with the appreciation of the multifactorial determinants of compliance, much of the most recent treatment literature still focuses on a simple one-dimensional approach to improving compliance rates (Epstein & Masek, 1978; Gabriel, Gagnon, & Bryon, 1977; Nessman, Carnahan, & Nugent, 1980).

Many previous treatment studies employing single-focus behavioral treatment report some positive behavior change but report brief, if any, follow-up (Barnes, 1976; Haynes, 1976; Ziezat, 1977). In our experience with such techniques, positive results frequently deteriorate as time passes. This failure to maintain long-term effect was seen in a recent study with diabetics. Wing et al. (1984) using a behavior modification approach (e.g., self-monitoring, exercise, monetary reward) toward increasing dietary compliance in diabetics found no significant treatment effect on weight loss at 16-month follow-up. They conclude that the techniques used to increase dietary change in the nonchronically ill obese may not be appropriate for chronically ill patients. They suggest that treatment approaches specific to the unique needs of the chronically ill patient need to be developed. The life experience of the chronically ill patient is unique and, as such, the application of a behavioral technology to increase compliance will often fail without incorporating recognition of these unique needs into any potential treatment plan.

Barofsky et al. (1978) argue that traditional behavioral approaches ignore a critical aspect of patienthood—quality of life—which greatly influences the degree of compliant behavior, particularly in long-term chronic illness. Quality of life includes

the varied social, cultural, familial, economic, and phenomenological consequences of compliance. In one of Barofsky's (1978)
first studies examining the relationship between quality of life
and compliance, sarcoma patients who discontinued chemotherapy or radiation treatment (31.1 percent of all protocol
patients) stated that their nonparticipation was due to the adverse
effect of the treatment on their daily lives. Although Barofsky
does not devalue informational or behavioral interventions for increasing compliance, he concludes that outcome variables—quality
of life after treatment—exerts a more significant impact on whether patients comply with medical recommendation. Research
involving techniques that increase compliance for a short period
of time would probably not gauge the life consequences of such
behavior changes for a credible enough period of time. Thus,
the impact on a family (and the family impact on the patient)
of dietary changes made by the hemodialysis patient need to be
measured not by the successful implementation of dietary changes
for a few weeks or a month but over a considerable amount of
time, a period that could be said to constitute a change in lifestyle.
The chapters in this book attempt to widen the notion of how
becoming more compliant with medical recommendation affects
the patient's life and how much knowledge can improve the
medical professional's interaction with the chronically ill patient.

THE COPING PROCESS AND NONCOMPLIANCE

The research of Lazarus and his colleagues serves as critical background to understanding how chronically ill patients cope with
medical recommendation. In a recent work, Cohen and Lazarus
(1979) concluded that coping and health outcome reflects
value-laden judgments about what constitutes health adaptation and "appropriate" patient behavior. In analyzing the
field of adherence to medical regimen, Lazarus notes that the
frequently cited low adherence rates are a function of a clinical environment that ignores, among other issues, the emotional life of patients. Through the interpretation and evaluation of the significance of their illness, patients may come to view
somatic health as one outcome value among many other values

that they might adopt. Medical staff project their values as the ultimate ones far outweighing other unique concerns of their patients (see Chapters 5 and 8). Rather than adopting the values promoted by professional health caretakers, patients' coping patterns may have several adaptational outcomes among which may be somatic health or greater satisfaction with daily life. The case of B.G., described in Chapter 5, illustrates how patients may choose to be noncompliant in favor of maintaining emotional equilibrium and stable family functioning.

The literature on coping with illness has overemphasized those threats and stresses directly related to the disease itself. Although researchers have demonstrated the multiple stresses that are precipitated by illness and affect other emotional and cognitive states, these factors have often been ignored or dismissed as of secondary importance by medical staff. Cohen and Lazarus (1979) summarize stresses affecting one's ability to cope with illness and how these stresses influence compliance levels by affecting lifelong belief systems, future plans, family relationship patterns, social roles, and self-concept, which may be perceived as equally critical to the patient as the physical threat of his illness and its sequelae. These personal matters may infringe more negatively on the patient's life than do the negative effects of noncompliance. Thus, Barofsky's (1978) notion of quality of life discussed above becomes a critical consideration in understanding noncompliant behavior.

In dialysis patients, for example, dietary abuse—clearly evidenced by biochemical analysis—may have no negative or very subtle negative consequences for the patient. The maintenance of emotional equilibrium, however, which may precipitate avoidance of dietary rules, often has significant motivational impetus. We saw such a case with a middle-aged dialysis patient from Samoa whose dietary compliance was clearly secondary to strong cultural values that equated being overweight with power and respect. Dietary restriction, though perhaps lessening physical discomfort at some future point, produced immediate emotional stress related to upsetting social roles critical to maintenance of an adequate self-concept.

Cohen and Lazarus (1979) view positive coping with chronic illness as a function of certain adaptive tasks precipitated by life changes due to the illness. It is instructive to review these five adaptive tasks:

1. Neutralize harmful environmental conditions (compliance with medical regime would be included here)
2. Adjust to negative events that result from the illness (i.e., limitations and changes)
3. Maintain self-image, through renewed sense of self-sufficiency
4. Maintain social relationships, including family and friends
5. Maintain emotional equilibrium, coping with feelings of anxiety, depression

Thus, the process of coping with chronic illness includes a number of substantial life adjustments, only one of which directly involves compliance with medical recommendations. Four other adaptive tasks include matters not necessarily related to and, possibly diametrically opposed to, regimen adherence. Individual variability in interpreting the meaning of illness and in the coping mechanisms used to deal with the effects of illness further complicates the reactions to illness. The assumption that one of these tasks is more important or more valuable than any other reflects values of those individuals setting institutional research priorities. The view of Lazarus and his colleagues about the complexity of what behaviors and attitudes define coping reinforce the multidetermined perspective on compliance which the authors within this volume support.

Thus, the editors of this volume espouse a multicause, multieffect model of compliant behavior in the chronically ill. We view compliance as resulting from the interplay of several domains of variables, including personal and environmental resources, life stressors, and the patient's appraisal and response to specific events within a particular life stage. Chapter topics have been chosen that are relevant to these domains and their interrelationships. The clinical implications of this framework for evaluating the relative effectiveness of treatment interventions and clarifying the determinants of their effectiveness are considered throughout the book.

As we conceptualize the compliance problem as multidimensional and complex—particularly in the context of the individual with severe chronic disease—we eschew the compliance technology proposed by a number of authors (Haynes, 1976; Zifferblatt, 1975). Compliance is more than the absence of appropriate behaviors which can be effectively produced through various educational and behavioral strategies. The clinical tactic with the chronically ill noncompliant patient must reflect this multidimensional view. Treatment strategies must be multifocused. We emphasize, then, the realities of compliance in the actual clinic environment seeing little benefit, at this stage, to focus on the narrow laboratory analogue. As Davidson (1976) suggested, only through the examination of the individual's experiencing the illness and demonstrating the noncompliance with the recommended regimen can we truly begin to understand the complexities and paradoxes of the noncompliant individual.

BIBLIOGRAPHY

Barnes, M. Token economy control of fluid overload in a patient receiving hemodialysis. *Journal of Behavior Therapy and Experimental Psychiatry, 7,* 305–306, 1976.

Barofsky, I. Compliance, adherence and the therapeutic alliance: Steps in the development of self-care. *Social Science and Medicine, 12,* 369–376, 1978.

Becker, M. The health belief model and personal health behavior. *Health Education Monographs, 2,* 324–473, 1974.

Becker, M. H., & Maiman, L. A. Sociobehavioral determinants of compliance with health and medical care recommendations. *Medical Care, 13,* 10–24, 1975.

Bloom, N., Cerkoney, K., & Hart, L. The relationship between the health beliefs model and compliance of persons with diabetes mellitus. *Diabetes Care, 3,* 490–500, 1980.

Burish, T., & Bradley, L. *Coping with chronic disease.* New York: Academic Press, 1983.

Cohen, F., & Lazarus, R. S. Coping with the stresses of illness. In G. C. Stone, F. Cohen, & N. E. Adler (Eds.), *Health psychology: A handbook.* San Francisco: Jossey-Bass, 1979.

Davidson, P. Therapeutic compliance, *Canadian Psychological Review, 17,* 247–259, 1976.

DiMatteo, M. R., & DiNicola, D. D. *Achieving patient compliance.* New York: Pergamon Press, 1982.

Epstein, L. H., & Cluss, P. A. A behavioral medicine perspective on adherence to long-term medical regimens. *Journal of Consulting and Clinical Psychology, 50,* 950-971, 1982.

Epstein, L. H. & Masek, B. Behavioral control of medical compliance. *Journal of Applied Behavioral Analysis, 11,* 1-10, 1978.

Foote, A., & Erfurt, J. Controlling hypertension: A cost-effective model. *Preventive Medicine, 6,* 319-343, 1977.

Fordyce, W., Fowler, R., & DeLateur, B. An application of behavior modification technique to a problem of chronic pain. *Behavior Research and Therapy, 6,* 105-107, 1968.

Gabriel, M., Gagnon, J., & Bryan, C. Improved patient compliance through use of a daily drug chart. *American Journal of Public Health, 67,* 968-969, 1977.

Haynes, R. B. A critical review of the "determinants" of patient compliance with therapeutic regimes. In D. L. Sackett & R. B. Haynes (Eds.), *Compliance with therapeutic regimes.* Baltimore: Johns Hopkins University Press, 1976.

Johnson, A., Taylor, D., Sackett, D., Dunnett, C. & Shinizu, S. Self-recording of BP in the management of hypertension. *Canadian Medical Association Journal, 119,* 1034-1039, 1978.

Kaplan De-Nour, A. Staff–patient interaction. In Norman B. Levy (Ed.), *PsychoNephrology II.* New York: Plenum Medical Book Company, 1983.

Kasl, S. V. Issues in patient adherence to health care regimens, *Journal of Human Stress, 1,* 5-17, 1975.

Kirscht, J., & Rosenstock, I. Patients' problems in following recommendations of health experts. In G. C. Stone, F. Cohen, & N. E. Adler (Eds.), *Health Psychology: A handbook.* San Francisco: Jossey-Bass, 1979.

Mazur, F. T. Adherence to health care regimens. In L. Pradley & C. Prokop (Eds.), *Medical psychology; Contributions to behavioral medicine.* New York: Academic Press, 1981.

McKenney, J., Slining, J., Henderson, H., Devins, D., & Barr, M. The effect of clinical pharmacy services on patients with essential hypertension. *Circulation, 48,* 1104-1111, 1973.

Minuchin, S. *Families and family therapy.* Cambridge: Harvard University Press, 1974.

Nessman, D., Carnahan, J., & Nugent, C. Increasing compliance: Patient operated hypertension groups. *Archieves of Internal Medicine, 140,* 1427-1430, 1980.

Sackett, D. L. The magnitude of compliance and noncompliance. In D. L. Sackett & R. B. Haynes (Eds.), *Compliance with therapeutic regimes.* Baltimore: Johns Hopkins University Press, 1976.

Sackett, D. L., & Haynes, R. B. *Compliance with therapeutic regimes.* Baltimore: Johns Hopkins University Press, 1976.

Schwartz, G. Testing the biopsychosocial model: The ultimate challenge facing behavioral medicine?, *Journal of Consulting and Clinical Psychology, 50,* 1040-1053, 1982.

Stone, G. Patient compliance and the role of expert. *Journal of Social Issues, 35,* 34-60, 1979.

Stone, G. C., Cohen, F., & Adler, N. E. (Eds.) *Health psychology: A handbook.* San Francisco: Jossey-Bass, 1979.

Tagliacozzo, D., & Ima, K. Knowledge of illness as a predictor of patient behavior. *Journal of Chronic Diseases, 22,* 765-775, 1970.

Tagliacozzo, D., Ima, K., & Lashof, J. Influencing the chronically ill: The role of prescriptions in premature separations of outpatient care. *Medical Care, 11,* 21-29, 1973.

Viney, L. L., & Westbrook, M. T. Psychological reactions to chronic illness— Related disability as a function of its severity and type. *Journal of Psychosomatic Research, 25,* 513-523, 1981.

Watkins, J., Williams, T., Martin, D., Hogan, M., & Anderson, E. A study of diabetic patients at home. *American Journal of Public Health, 57,* 452-459, 1967.

Weiss, S. Health psychology: The time is now, *Health Psychology, 1,* 81-92, 1982.

Williams, T. F., Martin, D., Hogan, M., Watkins, J., & Ellis, E. The clinical picture of diabetic control in four settings. *American Journal of Public Health, 57,* 441-451, 1967.

Wing, R., Epstein, L., & Nowalk, M. Dietary adherence in patients with diabetes. *Behavioral Medicine Update, 6,* 17-22, 1984.

Witenberg, S., Blanchard, E., McCoy, G., Suls, J., & McGoldrick, M. Evaluation of compliance in home and center hemodialysis patients. *Health Psychology, 2,* 227-239, 1983.

Yalom, I. *Existential psychotherapy.* New York: Basic Books, 1980.

Zaner, R. Dialysis and ethics: Be strong and trust (please!). In Norman Levy (Ed.), *PsychoNephrology I.* New York: Plenum Medical Book Company, 1981.

Ziezat, H. Behavior modification in the treatment of hypertension. *International Journal of Psychiatry in Medicine, 8,* 257-265, 1977.

Zifferblatt, S. M. Increasing patient compliance through applied analysis of behavior. *Preventative Medicine, 4,* 173-182, 1975.

3

Noncompliance as Indirect Self-Destructive Behavior

Norman L. Farberow

Problems of compliance and noncompliance have been noted in the records of medicine men and men of medicine since the earliest of times (Davidson, 1976). They were not always of equal concern, however, for the therapeutic procedures in succeeding eras provided wide differences in opportunity for noncompliance. Before the Renaissance, Davidson (1976) points out, treatment methods did not require compliance from the patient. Rather, methods, which included such treatments as bloodletting and leeching, were imposed on the patient, even against his will if necessary.

It was essentially when drugs were developed in the 19th century, along with slowly increasing recognition of individual rights, that noncompliance began to appear as a medical problem. The patient was gradually being entrusted more often with his own care, and the faithfulness with which he carried out the prescriptions of the doctor often determined the rate at which he improved or the amount of time elapsing before his death.

Davidson lists a number of studies that searched for factors related to compliance without success, such as demographic, illness, attitudes toward the doctor, illness, and death, and personality measures, e.g., projective tests, locus of control, and others. However, he says, one good reason for the lack of success and the disparity in results may well have been the variety of definitions for compliance and noncompliance that have been used. In this chapter, noncompliance is restricted to medical noncompliance in a chronic illness, in which the prescriptions and recommendations of the physician for self-care are ignored, contradicted, even flouted, and negative results, actual or potential, are disregarded or denied. Such actions and attitudes are viewed as indirect self-destructive behaviors.

INDIRECT SELF-DESTRUCTIVE BEHAVIORS

It is only recently that the study of suicide has broadened its area of concern to include noncompliant behavior. This has been possible with the delineation of a number of behaviors as indirectly self-destructive, differentiating them from direct self-destructive behaviors and exploring their similarities, differences, characteristics, and parameters. These explorations have found that medical noncompliant behaviors made up a large number of indirect self-destructive behaviors. Others included the addictions, violence, accident proneness, crime and delinquency, excessive risk-taking, compulsive gambling, and philosophies of self-denial.

The concept of indirect self-destructive behavior has actually been recognized for many years, but has not, except for some notable exceptions, been developed. Durkheim (1897), for example, viewed it as a sort of embryonic suicide but, having noted and recognized it, confined his studies to the published factual data of certified (overt) suicide deaths. Meerloo (1968) called it hidden suicide, Blachly (1973) coined the term "seduction," and Shneidman (1968) used the term "subintentioned." None, however, conducted any systematic or controlled investigations of the behaviors. Karl Menninger (1938) was the true pioneer in developing the concept, identifying what he called focal suicide and organic suicide as examples of the way in which a person used his body against himself, bringing about severe self-injury and often hastening his own death. Menninger found these forms of indirect self-destructive behaviors necessary to understand the full range of suicidal activity and to illustrate the interactions in his theory of the basic motivational elements in suicide: the wish to kill, the wish to be killed, and the wish to die. These three elements, he theorized, are always present but are expressed in different degrees in the interaction of the life and death instincts.

It is primarily the factor of intention which differentiates between the major categories of direct and indirect suicide. Intention is present in direct suicide and absent in indirect suicide. Intention exists on a continuum from full to none, and it is at the point along the continuum that intention for death or self-injury disappears from consciousness that the self-destructive behaviors become indirect. Awareness of the potential of death or self-injury may be present, but there is no intention that either shall occur. In many of the activities, the behavior does not have an immediate effect so that the result is slow and cumulative. Awareness of the long-range effects may be denied, or more often, the person does not care. Thus, temporal and awareness aspects in the behavior supplement the factor of intention in differentiating direct and indirect self-destructive behavior.

Indirect self-destructive behavior (ISDB) appears in a wide range of behaviors and conditions (Farberow, 1980). A convenient classification of ISDB is determined by the primary impact of the ISDB on either the body or social/personal status and on whether or not a prior physical condition exists.

In the first row of Table 3.1, where a prior chronic illness or long-term physical condition exists, the individual's ISDB may seriously affect the illness or the conditions, bringing injury, loss of limb, deteriorating functions, and even premature death. Thus, in hypertension, continued work in highly stressful occupations or disregard of diet requirements will keep the blood pressure up. Continued smoking in Buerger's disease and cardiorespiratory illnesses will endanger the circulatory capacity remaining. The reader will readily recognize these as medical noncompliant behaviors. Some persons are unable to adapt to the loss of a limb or the senses of sight or hearing and withdraw in bitterness and resentment. While not medical noncompliance, their actions effectively negate their social and personal lives and qualify as indirect self-destructive behaviors.

In the second row of the table, where no prior illness or physical condition exists, the activity itself becomes the ISDB, with either actual or potential damage to the body and/or to the self. The addictions appear in the first group, with abuse of food, tobacco, drugs, and alcohol serving as the ISDB actually debilitating

TABLE 3.1 Indirect Self-Destructive Behavior

	Primary Effect on	
Prior Physical Condition	Body	Person
Present:		
Prior physical condition exists: individual's activity increases actual or potential damage	Psychosomatic: asthma, ulcer, colitis, dermatitis, etc. Diabetes Buerger's, Raynaud's diseases Cardiorespiratory diseases Hypertension Physical debilities of elderly Invalidism Polysurgery Neurasthenia Hypochondria Malingering Nephritis/hemodialysis	Loss of body part or function: limb (accident), mobility (stroke, aging), mastectomy sequelae, sensory loss (blindness, deafness)
Absent:	*Actual:*	*Actual:*
No prior physical condition exists; actual or potential damage may result from activity	Hyperobesity Smoking Drug addiction Alcoholism Self-mutilation	Severe sexual disorders Asceticism
	Potential:	*Potential:*
	Violent crime; rioting Assassination Repeated accidents; traffic, industrial	Nonviolent crime, delinquency, compulsive gambling
	Stress-seeking, risk-taking Mountain climbing Sports parachuting or skydiving Scuba diving Hang-gliding Circus artists, trapeze performers Stuntmen Motorcycle, boat and auto racing Violent contact sports (boxing)	*Stress-seeking, risk-taking* Games of risk, chance Stock market speculation

From Norman L. Farberow, *The Many Faces of Suicide,* p. 19. Reprinted with persion from the McGraw-Hill Book Company. Copyright © 1980.

the body, and criminal activity and accident proneness acting as
the potential self-injurious behaviors. Sexual disorders and asceti-
cism affect the self negatively in this group, while nonviolent
crime and compulsive gambling have the potential for harm to the
person and his social functioning.

A third row consists of activities within those sports and
occupations that have high elements of risk both to life and limb
and to social status and position. These activities occupy special
positions for it is their quality or risk which makes them attractive for many reasons. Society tends to tolerate and even to ad-
mire the participants in such behaviors, perhaps enjoying by
proxy the skirting with danger and the explorations into the unknown. By themselves, the activities are dangerous and even
addictive (Delk, 1980; Hartung & Farge, 1983), but generally
every effort is made by the participant to foresee and forestall
the danger. It is when the participant ignores, disregards, and
flouts the known dangers that the risks taken become self-destructive.

Noncompliance obviously plays a role in each of the groups,
whether through ignoring safety procedures in the high-risk
sports or the admonitions of dangers in the addictions. Our
greatest concern with noncompliance occurs in the medical
conditions (row 1 of Table 3.1) where, primarily in chronic
illnesses, the individual uses the opportunities provided by his
long-term illness to harm or injure himself, to worsen his condition needlessly, and in some instances, to bring about an early
death.

STUDIES OF NONCOMPLIANT ISDB

A number of studies of ISDB in chronic illnesses have been conducted by the author. These can be summarized briefly.

Diabetes Mellitus

This exploratory study (Farberow, Stein, Darbonne, & Hirsch,
1970a) was aimed at determining whether ISDB appeared as a
characteristic pattern in some chronically ill patients, and if so,

what were its predominant features. The study compared the records of 24 male experimental subjects and 24 matched controls, with the experimental patients defined as having been admitted to the hospital at least three times because of diabetic acidosis or insulin coma, conditions that could be taken as prima facie evidence of disregard or neglect of their illness. In the experimental group, the average number of admissions for diabetics out of control was eight while for the controls and a baseline group (all diabetic patients discharged from a hospital in one year) the average was less than two. The differences between the experimental and the control groups in this respect indicate how much greater a problem the experimentals present for hospital administration. The average length of illness for the two groups and for the baseline group was nearly 10 years. The uncooperative diabetics also tended to have many more related (to diabetes) and unrelated illnesses. The experimental group tended to be younger than the baseline population and included significantly more single, separated, or divorced patients, implying difficulties in establishing and maintaining interpersonal relationships. The experimental patient was described in the records as uncooperative because he flouted hospital rules, disregarded diet regulations and medical prescriptions, failed appointments, and made unending demands. In contrast, the cooperative patients were considered to be friendly, quiet, and sociable.

The experimental group showed primarily denial and negligence in their attitudes toward their illness. They were also highly dependent persons and openly demanded that they be taken care of. Their remarks showed that they considered their illness the hospital's responsibility, not theirs. The most frequent descriptive phrases for the experimental group referred to passivity, dependency, hostility, and antisocial behavior. They were also inclined to be suspicious, impulsive, and complaining, and drinking continued to be a problem for most. In contrast, the controls were seen as passive-dependent, anxious, depressed, but also quiet or cheerful and pleasant. The experimental group showed more prior overt suicidal behavior as well as more indirect self-destructive behavior than the controls.

A further study of 12 uncooperative patients by means of the Rorschach test substantiated their low frustration tolerance, poor impulse control, and anxiety frequently accompanied by agitation (Farberow, Darbonne, Stein, & Hirsch, 1970b). There seemed to be two subgroups. In the first, the illness seemed to play no dynamically meaningful role in the patient's behavior, but rather the illness was exacerbated as a concomitant of impulse-gratifying activities. In the second, the illness seemed to have been integrated into defensive personality patterns where it was deliberately manipulated for personal satisfaction. An ability to use massive denial in a number of the patients allowed strong tendencies for impulse gratification to seek expression. The other side of the coin was a minimal tolerance for frustration or delay. There also seemed to be little, if any, future orientation or concern.

Buerger's Disease

A second study focused on patients with diagnoses of thrombo-angiitis obliterans, or Buerger's disease (Farberow & Nehemkis, 1979). Buerger's illness seems to be differentiated from diabetes in that it is more specifically related and controlled by a single activity, smoking. Diabetes is more systemic and complicated in terms of control, requiring more than just insulin or diet alone, and other personality factors may therefore fashion subsequent behavior more variably.

The study was also conducted in two parts, with the first part examining case files of matched identified cooperative and uncooperative Buerger's disease patients; and the second an in-depth study of patients currently in the hospital using interview and psychological test data, such as a Time Metaphor Test, Futurity Scale, and the Rorschach. In order to specify more clearly the characteristics of ISDB, all of the experimental group patients were identified as uncooperative as judged by a medical consultant, on the basis of neglect of medical advice, refusing to abstain or markedly reduce cigarette smoking, not avoiding contact with cold, and resisting hospital regimen. For example, in the hospital a patient refused physical therapy or was reluctant to exercise related muscles after amputation, or avoided practice with his prosthesis. He was querulous, demanding, and annoying to other patients; insisted on instant relief from pain; and frequently neglected accompanying medical conditions. Matched controls were selected with the criteria that the patient did observe his prescribed medical regimen, abstained or markedly reduced his smoking, changed his geographical location to a warmer climate, and even changed his profession to help his medical condition. In the hospital, he observed regulations and seemed eager to be rehabilitated.

Each group consisted of 26 patients, and both groups were compared with a total sample of all Buerger's cases discharged from the hospital during a subsequent year, consisting of 25 cases. The modal description of the uncooperative Buerger's patient showed him to be around 50 years of age, to have had Buerger's disease for approximately 15 years, and to have an average of five additional illnesses that complicated his treatment program. He was likely to be married and to function in a skilled level job when not in the hospital. He tended to minimize his illness and to place the responsibility for his treatment on the hospital. Most significant in his attitude toward his illness was that he refused to give up smoking despite being told that this was the major avenue for arresting the disease. In contrast, the cooperative Buerger patient gave up smoking entirely or at least markedly reduced the amount. The uncooperative Buerger patient continued to drink fairly heavily and to accumulate a number of drunk-driving arrests. In the hospital, he hindered his own care by getting into fights and frequently wound up with disciplinary discharges. He refused to submit to necessary examinations.

The psychological tests and interview material indicated that the uncooperative Buerger patient did not value time nor was he invested in production and achievement goals esteemed in our society. He seemed less driven and without ambition to achieve distant goals. He hated the prospects of a dull life, apparently preferring the excitement and pleasures of the here-and-now to the promises of a future. The uncooperative Buerger patient did not describe feelings of helplessness or hopelessness. Helplessness seems to be derived from the feelings of loss of control and inability to do anything about his situation personally. However, this patient appeared instead to have found a mechanism for maintaining control that was highly effective and frequently gratifying. Thus, the Buerger's ISDB patient was found infrequently to be depressed. With the patient's lesser investment in relationships with others and in future goals, defeats were not seen as evidence of inadequacy; they were merely temporary setbacks in the pursuit of pleasure from the moment. Almost incredibly, too, loss of a limb or function or sense were temporary discomforts that simply occurred and were to be endured.

Elderly Chronically Ill

This study of predominantly elderly patients who were chronically ill and in either a nursing home or on a long-term hospital ward differed from the previous researches in ISDB in that the focus was on patients who exhibited a wide range of illnesses, not one specific illness (Nelson & Farberow, 1980). The major types of illnesses found in these patients were carcinomas, cerebral vascular accidents, and respiratory diseases. The average length of stay for a patient on the ward was 1½ years, and the typical patient was described as "poor, isolated, and having no place to go." The population in terms of sex (male), age (elderly), health (poor), and available resources (few or none) seemed to represent a high suicide-risk population. However, the overt suicidal behavior was minimal, which led to the question of whether or not their multiple illnesses also provided them with the means and opportunity to use indirect self-destructive behavior as a suicide substitute.

A scale was constructed for observers to rate the frequency of ISDB. The scale was constructed by using behaviors described in the literature, from previous studies, and from suggestions from members of a hospital intermediate care ward staff. The final scale consisted of 56 behaviors grouped under categories of eating (refusing food, eating proscribed foods, etc.), drinking (alcohol, drinking liquids not permitted, not drinking, etc.), smoking (against medical advice, in unauthorized places, etc.), abuse of medication (refusing, taking unauthorized medications, illicit drugs, etc.), interaction with other patients (stealing, verbal abuse, etc.), interaction with staff (refusing to follow doctors' and nurses' orders, verbal abuse of staff, etc.), abuse of treatment program or hospital policy (refusing treatment, staying in bed all day against medical advice, leaving hospital against medical advice, etc.), and self-injury (scratching excessively, pulling off bandages and dressings, etc.).

A patient interview schedule was developed that incorporated a number of psychological tests and that obtained information on previously determined pertinent variables, such as locus of control, rigidity, life satisfaction, risk-taking, manipulativeness, suicide potential, and sense of futurity. A total of 58 patients were rated, of whom 53 completed all or portions of the interview. Patients were rated for their ISDB over a seven-day period by the nursing staff on their wards. After they were rated, their attending physicians evaluated the relative harmfulness of each observed behavior for each patient and then completed a staff interview schedule on each.

The results of this study showed that, in descending order of significance, the most important correlates of ISDB among the elderly chronically ill were the number and intensity of the personal losses experienced, such as health, loved ones, and independence; dissatisfaction with the hospital; little satisfaction from life; a positive orientation toward risk-taking; and a tendency toward a higher suicide potential. In addition, there was a high level of manipulativeness, fatalism, and a lack of contact with persons outside the hospital. There was a high inverse correlation between suicide potential and life satisfaction, which leads to the inference that ISDB among the elderly chronically ill is generated by feelings of isolation and loss, variables which also are known to produce direct suicidal behavior. The extent of religious involvement also appears to limit the use of ISDB to handle depression and frustration in much the same way that it inhibits the occurrence of direct suicidal behavior.

One possible use of ISDB by the elderly chronically ill may be as a matter of convenience, for through such behavior the chronically ill patient has at his disposal a form of behavior that avoids the stigma and the taboos that characterize overt suicide. Also, the extent to which ISDB frustrates the hospital staff may explain the use of ISDB by some patients as a vehicle for expressing dissatisfaction with their own mastery of the institutional environment.

Hyperobese

A group of hyperobese (N=25), average weight 327 pounds, who were applying to a hospital for a jejunoileostomy, was compared with overtly self-destructive persons who had attempted suicide (N=28) (Farberow & Williams, in press). Measuring instruments consisted of Cattell's 16 personality factor inventory (i.e., 16 PF) and a questionnaire combining established scales with questions of special interest. Concepts tested were related to feelings of self-value, sense of adequacy and self-control, futurity, and excitement-seeking.

The average hyperobese in this study was a 43-year-old Caucasian married man who generally had a variety of metabolic and nutritional illnesses and the psychiatric syndrome of depression. However, he assumed control of his own life, planned ahead, and was hopeful his plans would work out. He felt powerless most often in relationships with spouse or lover and felt little appreciation from society or neighbors. He would prefer to be dead if he had a fatal disease, if he were a severe financial burden to his family, or if his death would help save another person's life. The hyperobese patient also tended to be relatively self-sufficient, independent-minded, and unconcerned about social approval. He seemed to feel a large gap between real and ideal self.

In the four concept areas used for focused comparisons, the hyperobese were differentiated from the attempted suicides, regarding themselves more positively, more adequate, and more future-oriented. However, they were not more stress-seeking than the attempted suicides.

Renal Hemodialysis Patients

A study was conducted with a group of 32 chronic renal hemodialysis patients for those characteristics of ISDB that had emerged as most salient in earlier studies: self-esteem, locus of control, flexibility and rigidity, impulsivity, futurity, risk-taking, and denial (Gerber, Farberow, Nehemkis, & Williams, 1981). The average age of the (all male) subjects was 52 years with a range of 31 to 80 years of age. Half the group were Caucasian, 75 percent were married, most had completed high school, and 53 percent were currently unemployed. Nearly half the patients had been on dialysis 3 to 4 years or longer, primarily for chronic nephritis and renal sclerosis. Most had secondary and tertiary illnesses as well. For resources and supports the patient turned most often to spouses, then children, siblings, friends, and fellow patients. Practically all the patients felt the hospital to be a strong source of support.

Ratings of cooperativeness were obtained from head nurse, physician, dietician, technician, and staff nurse based on care of the blood access, observance of appointments, taking of medication, reporting changes in physical conditions, limiting of physical activities as directed by staff, likeableness, cooperativeness compared with other patients, and concern shown for own general welfare and health. The group was divided into two subgroups on the basis of an average of the ratings as more versus less cooperative patients, and the demographic, medical, and psychological data from the two groups were compared. The findings suggested that the less cooperative hemodialysis patients had experienced the illness as a more severe blow to their self-concept and had failed to integrate their illness into an effective, adaptive life pattern. The uncooperative patients felt less valued and less appreciated not only by their family but also by neighbors and by hospital staff. They showed significantly more anger and withdrawal than the cooperative group and appeared to have compensated for a significantly greater sense of powerlessness by the development of manipulative behaviors in relating to their medical caretakers.

Case File Study

The studies outlined above have focused on personality attributes and dynamics of ISDB users. The purpose of the file case survey, however, was different, in that its primary objective was to obtain information on the occurrence and distribution of ISDB in five treatment groups: two drug rehabilitation programs, two hospital populations, and one youth delinquency program (Farberow & Nelson, 1980). The drug treatment programs consisted of a methadone maintenance group (N=200), in which clients were maintained on minimal dosages of methadone at the same time they were undergoing an outpatient rehabilitative program involving counseling, health care services, and occupational therapy; and a second drug rehabilitation group (N=287) of clients recently released from prison after serving a term for drug abuse or a related offense. The subjects were on parole, and the treatment was the same as for the methadone group except that it was drug free. A third group was made up of delinquent youth (*N*=301), ranging in age from 16 to 18, who had fallen into trouble with the law and who were diverted from criminal justice into rehabilitation programs providing counseling, tutorial, and recreational services. The remaining two groups were patients in Veterans Hospitals with either a primary neuropsychiatric diagnosis (*N*=764) or a primary medical or surgical diagnosis (*N*=249). While on the hospital rolls, these patients committed suicide. The total number of subjects in the study was 2,391. Although the records originally served different purposes than the aim of the study, it was possible to abstract each subject's file for indications of indirect self-destructive behavior.

ISDB was recorded in four main areas: in the form of noncompliance with the treatment program, alcohol abuse, drug abuse, and criminal behavior. Noncompliance with the treatment program was noted especially in terms of observation of medical regimen, taking medication as prescribed, making changes in life activities as recommended, keeping a prescribed diet, following hospital or agency regulations, and maintaining prescribed psychotherapy activities. Other forms of indirect self-destructive behavior were also noted, such as hyperobesity, anorexia, compulsive gambling, extreme withdrawal from social activity, frequent involvement in physical fights, sexual masochism, victimization, self-mutilation, and engaging in highly dangerous occupations and sports.

There was no difficulty in retrieving indirect self-destructive behavior from the records. Aside from the youth diversion group, evidence of each of the forms of ISDB was found in all the other groups. The youth diversion group had practically no references to the ISDB categories other than noncompliance with recommended changes in life activities and with prescribed therapy, drug abuse, social withdrawal, fighting, and delinquency. Apparently the other categories have not yet had a chance to apply in such areas as medical noncompliance and alcohol abuse. When the behavior in question is related to antisocial acting-out and self-abuse, there is as much evidence of ISDB in their records as in others. Age seems to increase the opportunity for physical and mental stress to appear and the possibility for the expression of ISDB tendencies through noncompliance to occur.

The methadone maintenance group was the greatest contributor to the ISDB scores, obtaining the highest score on noncompliance in such areas as medical regimen, making recommended changes in detrimental life activities, with prescribed physical and psychotherapy, and in nonspecified areas. One possible explanation for their high scores is that the members of the methadone group made fewer changes in an already self-destructive lifestyle than those in any of the other groups. The treatment program allowed them to continue to be drug dependent. Even though the dispensing of the methadone is rigidly controlled, there is undoubtedly much black market activity. The second drug rehabilitation group was much more motivated to be compliant since infractions could lead to their being returned to prison, and no substitute addictive drugs were used in their program.

The psychiatric patients were most frequently noncompliant with hospital or treatment group regulations and with not taking prescribed medications. The most frequent noncompliant behaviors for the general medical and surgical patients were not making the recommended changes in life activities and not following hospital regulations.

Alcohol was one of the most frequent forms of ISDB. It appeared in from one-half to one-third of the suicides and from one-third to one-fourth of the drug abusers. Even in the youth diversion group, 5 percent were already noted to be problem drinkers. About 20 percent were also known to be drug abusers.

Withdrawal from social activity was most often noted for the hospital groups. Violence was common in all the groups, especially the youth diversion group.

The relationship among different kinds of self-destructive behavior was examined. As expected, the two committed-suicide groups showed much prior suicidal behavior (attempts, threats), about 50 percent, and prior notations of feelings of helplessness, hopelessness, and worthlessness, about 45 percent. The drug groups also showed direct self-destructive behavior (attempts, threats), about 12 percent, but the methadone group showed much of the suicidal triad of feelings, about 22 percent. The youth diversion group showed no overt self-destructive behavior, but surprisingly, at least 10 percent had the triad of suicidal feelings.

In general, the hospital suicide groups showed high direct self-destructive behavior and moderate to low degrees of medical noncompliance. They also showed moderate to high violence, high alcohol abuse, and high withdrawal from social activities. The drug abuse groups showed low to moderate direct self-destructive behavior, low to moderate medical noncompliance, and moderate antisocial violent behaviors and alcohol abuse. The young people showed very little direct self-destructive behavior and practically no ISDB, except for fighting and some drug abuse.

The above listed studies now provide an outline of the salient characteristics of males who are most likely to engage in indirect self-destructive behavior, especially when they are living with a chronic illness that has required a variety of physical, personal, social, vocational, and sexual adaptations. Age apparently plays a general role insofar as ISDB seems to increase with age, with the elderly showing the greatest kind and number of ISDB (as well as direct suicidal behavior). Symptomatically, the results of neglect or disregard of the prescribed medical regimen produces physical symptoms characteristic of the illness, such as diabetic acidosis, insulin coma, circulatory distress, gangrene, excessive weight loss or gain, malnutrition, phenylketonuria, amputation, etc. Cognitive disturbance is rare, although reasoning seems shallow and superficial.

Dynamically, the motivation is directed toward gratification from present pleasures. Feelings of inadequacy are present but only moderately; most behaviors are oriented toward self, not others, and there is frequently poor social adjustment with many feelings of personal losses. Typically, the ISDB does not occur under conditions of great stress but rather when life seems smooth. One wonders whether life becomes a little too smooth, perhaps even boring, resulting in the characteristic need to stimulate excitement. Risk-taking lends meaning to existence; the attraction to gambling is more in the process than the outcome.

Future orientation is low, resulting in a hedonistic investment in the present and its current gratifications. Capacity for delay of gratification is minimal, and the behavior seems to occur with little or no immediate precipitating stress.

The most prominent coping mechanisms seem to be denial, narcissism, regression, and suppression. Relationships are likely to be casual and uninvested, a source of self-gratification rather than a mutual validational interaction.

Clinical Aspects

As with most human behaviors there are both positive and negative aspects of both compliant and noncompliant behavior in our society. A measurement of the distribution of noncompliant behaviors in the general population has never been made. One estimate is that the numbers of those who are frequently or intensively noncompliant would probably be small and the numbers of those who are rarely noncompliant would probably be large. While our society values innovation and independence, it insists for the most part on compliance with its rules, regulations, laws, mores, and manners. Most persons, in other words, learn to value society's approval and to be observant of rules and regulations, considerate of requirements for social and personal functioning, and courteous and polite in recognition of others' needs. We usually consider noncompliant behavior, especially when it is high or extreme in expression, as negative and the people in whom it appears as emotionally immature, psychologically and socially less developed, and even emotionally disturbed. In such persons, noncompliance has undesirable consequences both for the individual and for society.

However, as with noncompliance, there are also aspects of compliance when it too becomes excessive that have been identified as negative. Excessive compliance manifested as obedience to authority at the expense of personal ethics is unique to no one age or nation (Rosenbaum, 1983, p. 45). At the extreme, compliance becomes conformity. Battegay (1983) warns that we have to start early to teach the dangers inherent in collective conformity, for the price paid for that state is individual freedom. As he points out, there are many forces pressing toward conformity in our society. Even our genetic code represents a certain degree of compulsion, and the early experience of childhood plus the demands of society, community, and culture can add to this relatively weak deterministic force to produce a highly undesirable social cloning. Some governments have fostered conformity as a means of control. Totalitarian societies are obvious examples, but additional societies based on religious tenets also are known. For example, Back (1983) reports a principle developed by Islamic mystics called "ketman," which accepted compliance for compliance's sake. The mystics decided that mystical knowledge was only for enlightened persons and should not be given to the multitude. Ideas were to be shared only with other enlightened people with whom it was safe to talk (p. 52). Pattison (1983) emphasizes that religion is the strongest force in human history around which norms of social organization are crystallized: ". . . religious compliance can be a force for human good or for inhuman destruction" (p. 134).

One of the most perverse forms of unhealthy compliance is found in cults wherein a brainwashed allegiance is demanded by a leader who is often emotionally ill but who is able through an oversimplification of life and personal needs to obtain a relinquishing of personal identity and a slavish subservience. Jones and his Peoples' Temple followers in Guyana is probably the most tragic example of just such extreme compliance.

Compliance, of course, also has its positive aspects. For Braun (1983), positive compliance indicates adaptive strength and a facility to bend with pressure or to cope with external reality without breaking personal codes or beliefs. Adaptive compliance, he says, reflects such qualities as tolerance, flexibility, eclecticism, openness, and quiet wisdom. "Healthy compliance may be an act of commitment to and continuity with one's roots and personal history . . . . It may be one aspect of mature love" (p. 143). Braun also makes clear that external compliance needs to be evaluated in terms of the individual, for, paradoxically, it may actually represent a procedure for allowing genuine creativity, attention to priorities, and inner autonomy.

In the same way, Braun says, noncompliance must be examined thoroughly in the context of the individual, for both external and internal noncompliance may sometimes be loving, creative acts of the highest order. To the physician who is treating the chronically ill, it is sometimes hard to appreciate the non-compliant act of a desperately ill patient, especially when it runs the high risk of injury or even death. While there are many motivations underlying such acts, there seem to be two that are primary: a search for renewed identity and self-validation, and the introduction of excitement and mastery into a life that otherwise feels dull and no longer in control.

Clinically, a pervasive, invasive chronic illness clamps a huge, restraining hand upon the individual, forcing many changes physically and personally, sometimes far-reaching in lifestyle, sometimes moderate in diet and exercise. In one classic example, a gifted athlete who had been a near-star miler came back from war service wounded and unable to compete in running any longer. The therapy task was to help him to change his self-concept and to accept the fact that he would never be able to run competitively again. His occasional noncompliant behavior was readily seen as a strong protest against the fate that had robbed him of his dream. Many noncompliant acts are validational declarations of an inner core of self, indomitable and unconquered. To some degree they insist that the body, ravaged as it may be by disease or injury, is still personal and not a meaningless collection of fat, tissue, nervous system, and bones that has been taken over by the illness, by the medical profession, or by both.

The second form of noncompliant behavior is related to the risk-taking, excitement-seeking behavior, which in and of itself may be highly positive. From one point of view, it has been those persons willing to take high risks, often venturing into the unknown, who have contributed to the progress of science and the broaching of the limits of knowledge. Explorers into unknown lands, venturers into space, experimenters with cures for virulent diseases have often been persons "noncompliant" with the advice of others and the limitations of knowledge of their time. Such persons are lured by the excitement, the challenge, and the risk, which, when endured and overcome, are both gratifying and self-confirming. While it may be true that most medical noncompliance does not fall into this positive sphere, for that portion that does, medicine should not only tolerate it but perhaps welcome it as a symptom of independence and potential creativity.

REFERENCES

Back, K. W. Compliance and conformity in an age of sincerity. In M. Rosenbaum (Ed.), *Compliant behavior*. New York: Human Sciences Press, 1983.

Battegay, R. Compliance? Between freedom and compulsion. In M. Rosenbaum (Ed.), *Compliant behavior*. New York: Human Sciences Press, 1983.

Blachly, P. H. *Seduction: A conceptual model in the drug dependencies and other contagious ills.* Springfield, IL: Charles C Thomas, 1973.

Braun, J. A. The healthy side of compliance. In M. Rosenbaum (Ed.), *Compliant behavior*. New York: Human Sciences Press, 1983.

Davidson, P. Therapeutic compliance. *Canadian Psychological Revue, 17(4),* 247–259, October 1976.

Delk, J. L. High risk sports as indirect self-destructive behavior. In N. L. Farberow (Ed.), *The many faces of suicide*. New York: McGraw-Hill, 1980.

Durkheim, E. *Suicide.* Glencoe, IL: Free Press, 1951. (Originally published, 1897)

Farberow, N. L. (Ed.). *The many faces of suicide*. New York: McGraw-Hill, 1980.

Farberow, N. L., Darbonne, A. R., Stein, K., & Hirsch, S. Self-destructive behavior of uncooperative diabetics. *Psychological Reports, 27,* 935–946, 1970b.

Farberow, N. L., & Nehemkis, A. M. Indirect self-destructive behavior in patients with Buerger's disease. *Journal of Personality Assessment, 43,* 86–96, 1979.

Farberow, N. L., & Nelson, F. L. Indirect self-destructive behaviors in drug abusers, suicidal and delinquency groups. (Final Report). Rockville, MD: National Institute of Drug Abuse, January 1980.

Farberow, N. L., Stein, K., Darbonne, A. R., & Hirsch, S. Indirect self-destructive behavior in diabetic patients. *Hospital Medicine, 6,* 123–135, 1970a.

Farberow, N. L., & Williams, J. L. Indirect self-destructive behavior and the hyperobese. In K. Achte (Ed.), *Research in Suicide, II.* Helsinki, Finland: *Psychiatrica Fennica,* 1985.

Gerber, K., Farberow, N. L., Nehemkis, A., & Williams, J. L. Indirect self-destructive behavior in chronic hemodialysis patients. *Suicide and Life-Threatening Behavior, 11*(1), 31–41, 1981.

Hartung, G. H., & Farge, E. J. Compulsive or excess sports. In S. J. Mule (Ed.), *Behavior in excess*. New York: Free Press, 1981.

Meerloo, J. A. M. Hidden suicide. In L. L. P. Resnik (Ed.), *Suicidal behaviors and management*. Boston, MA: Little, Brown, 1968.

Menninger, K. A. *Man against himself.* New York: Harcourt Brace, 1938.

Nelson, F. L., & Farberow, N. L. Indirect self-destructive behavior in the elderly nursing home patient. *Journal of Gerontology, 35*(6), 949–957, 1980.

Pattison, E. M. Religion and compliance. In Max Rosenbaum (Ed.), *Compliant behavior*. New York: Human Sciences Press, 1983.

Rosenbaum, M. (Ed.). *Compliant behavior.* New York: Human Sciences Press, 1983.
Shneidman, E. S. Orientations toward death: A vital aspect of the study of lives. In H. L. P. Resnik (Ed.), *Suicidal behaviors and Management.* Boston, MA: Little, Brown, 1968.

4

Adherence: A Cognitive-Behavioral Perspective

Dennis C. Turk
Peter Salovey
Mark D. Litt

INTRODUCTION

It has been claimed that the most cost-effective approach to the delivery of health care would involve increasing adherence to medically recommended regimens and healthy lifestyles (cf. Benfari, Eaker, & Stoll, 1981; Richmond, 1979). According to Dunbar and Stunkard (1979), however, rates of adherence are quite low: 20 to 50 percent of patients fail to appear for scheduled appointments, 20 to 80 percent make errors in taking medications, 25 to 60 percent stop taking medications prior to being instructed to do so, and 20 to 80 percent of patients drop out of various lifestyle change programs. Likewise, lifestyle changes are rarely maintained: up to 95 percent of weight-loss patients never achieve their ideal weight, and 75 percent of individuals who quit smoking begin anew within six months (Dunbar, 1980; Dunbar & Stunkard, 1979).

Two terms are often used to describe a patient's performance of medically or psychologically prescribed behaviors: compliance and adherence. Although compliance seems to connote conformity and acquiescence to the demands of a health care professional,

Support for this project was provided by a Veterans Administration Merit Review Grant and a Biomedical Research Support Grant NIH 5–507–RR7015.

adherence seems to suggest more self-motivated perseverance with a treatment regimen. In this chapter, consistent with the cognitive-behavioral emphasis on collaboration, active participation, and self-control, we will use the less authoritarian term of adherence.

The purpose of this chapter is not to review the various demographic, medical, personality, care-giver, and social psychological factors associated with adherence to therapeutic regimens. Such material has been reviewed elsewhere (cf. DiMatteo & DiNicola, 1980; Dunbar, 1980; Epstein & Cluss, 1982; Haynes, Taylor, & Sackett, 1979; Sackett & Haynes, 1976). Rather, we offer a cognitive-behavioral perspective on adherence, followed by some specific cognitive and behavioral techniques that have proven useful in increasing patient adherence.

Before offering our general perspective on adherence, however, we wish to sensitize the reader to several issues that have not received sufficient attention in the adherence literature. The first issue concerns the usual practice of treating adherence in a generic sense, as including *any* prescribed behavior presented by a health care professional. That is, when investigators and practitioners speak of adherence, they include a diversity of simple behaviors and complex therapeutic regimens ranging from keeping appointments (e.g., Tracy, 1977) and having a chest X-ray (Hochbaum, 1956) to refraining from alcohol, cigarettes, and high-caloric food for an extended period of time (e.g., Chaney, O'Leary, & Marlatt, 1978; Mahoney & Mahoney, 1976); taking antihypertension medication for many years (e.g., Steckel & Swain, 1977); limiting liquids, potassium, and taking potassium-binding medication (i.e., hemodialysis patients, Cummings, Becker, Kirscht, & Levin, 1981); and monitoring nutrient and caloric intake, urine and blood testing two to three times per day, taking medication, and monitoring exercise (i.e., diabetic patients, Speers & Turk, 1982). Examination of this list reveals the diversity and complexity of the volume of self-care behaviors. Classifying such types of adherence as obtaining a chest X-ray with the major lifestyle changes of diabetic and hemodialysis patients seems inappropriate. Strategies to improve adherence to relatively brief regimens may vary considerably from the strategies required for more chronic conditions.

A second problem in the adherence literature is the observation that many self-care regimens require multiple behaviors.

Adherence behaviors have been treated as unidimensional so that hemodialysis patients who adhere to taking their medication are assumed to be also controlling their fluid intake and controlling their diets. It is quite possible, however, that complex regimens may lead to differential adherence rates for different behaviors (e.g., Kirscht, Kirscht, & Rosenstock, 1981). There is little evidence to suggest that performing one self-care behavior will be associated with performing a second. Different individuals may be adherent to some behaviors and not others. Moreover, different approaches to increasing adherence may be necessary for different behaviors and for different individuals.

A final issue to note is the assumption that if patients are adherent to the self-care regimen, they *will* improve their health. The evidence is far from clear that this is the case. Frequently, patients improve despite low rates of adherence and at times do not get better despite high rates of adherence (Dunbar & Stunkard, 1979; Epstein & Cluss, 1982). Results such as these make it difficult to tell patients that if they fail to adhere, certain consequences will occur or that strict adherence will necessarily result in prevention of complications. Although the health care provider may not be able to guarantee that complications will be reduced if the patient adheres to the medical regimen, the potential consequences of nonadherence are sufficiently severe to warrant a cautious approach (i.e., performing self-care behaviors) rather than leaving it to fate.

In this chapter, we will focus on adherence to some of the most complex, demanding, and lengthy therapeutic regimens. Thus, we will emphasize self-care and self-control, by which we mean that patients need to assume major responsibility for the treatment of their condition or problem. Self-care and self-control imply that patients also need to engage in any of a number of behaviors related to maintenance of their health. Thus, when we use the term self-care, we are implicitly including a component of self-control.

A COGNITIVE-BEHAVIORAL MODEL OF ADHERENCE TO SELF-CARE REGIMENS

A cognitive-behavioral perspective primarily focuses on the underlying assumptions that guide behavior and how such assumptions are promoted by the way in which the individual constructs his or her world. The major theoretical underpinnings of this view, social-learning theory, holds that behavior is reciprocally determined by an individual's cognitive structures and processes, interpersonal behaviors, and their resulting consequences from the environment (Bandura, 1978; Meichenbaum & Turk, 1982; Turk & Speers, 1983). To change behaviors, interventions can be initiated at the point of cognitive structures (changing beliefs and meaning systems), cognitive processes (changing automatic thoughts, images, and coping skills), behavioral acts, and/or environmental characteristics and consequences (Turk & Salovey, 1983; Turk & Speers, 1983).

The components of the cognitive-behavioral model of adherence can be viewed as fitting into four general categories: knowledge and skills, beliefs, motivation, and actions (Speers & Turk, 1982). The present description is presented as a heuristic model that points out the complexities of adherence.

Adherence is an interactive process; more than one component is likely to affect behavior at any one time. Moreover, many of the components are interrelated and will influence each other as they affect the patient's behavior. For example, actions will influence subsequent motivation and beliefs. A breakdown or failure of any of the components may lead to nonadherence. After describing characteristics of these four components, we will consider approaches to addressing each, with the goal of increasing health care providers' skills in assisting patients to enhance adherence.

Knowledge and Skills

For satisfactory adherence, the patient needs to have appropriate knowledge about his or her disorder and information about the specific self-care behaviors required by the disorder. Knowing *what* to do may be inadequate if the patient does not know *how* to do it. For example, people with diabetes may know that before they eat a bowl of cereal, they should count the calories but may not know exactly how to do it. Diabetic patients need to know what types of food to eat (unsweetened cereal and low-fat milk), how to measure each quantity of food, and how to determine the number of calories in each quantity. In addition, understanding the need for adherence and the rationale for each specific self-care behavior is particularly important. Finally, the patient needs to have the skills (motoric and cognitive) necessary to carry out the self-care behaviors in a satisfactory manner. Consider the case of a diabetic with limited vision trying to discriminate small differences in color charts associated with home urine testing, or the diabetic with limited education trying to compute and balance food from different food groups as is usually suggested to be important for self-care.

Insufficient attention has been given by health care providers to internal processing of information. At the level of internal processing, patients need first to select and file the information in memory and then to retain it so that it can be used in future situations. Often patients report that they understand what to do after receiving instruction; however, when asked to perform the task, they err and report that they thought the health care provider said something different from what was actually presented (Ley, 1979). Even comprehending the information appropriately when immediately presented will not be sufficient if the patient forgets or distorts it shortly thereafter.

Cassata (1978) has summarized a number of findings related to information provided to patients by health care providers:

1. Patients forget much of what the doctor tells them.
2. Instructions and advice are more likely to be forgotten than other information.
3. The more a patient is told, the greater the proportion he or she will forget.
4. Patients will remember (a) what they are told first and (b) what they consider most important.
5. Intelligent patients do not remember more than less intelligent patients.
6. Older patients remember just as much as younger ones.
7. Moderately anxious patients recall more of what they are told than highly anxious patients or patients who are not anxious.
8. The more medical knowledge a patient has, the more he or she will recall.

9. If the patient writes down what the doctor says, he or she will remember it just as well as if he or she merely hears it. (p. 498)

It may be necessary for patients to rehearse the information mentally and mechanically so that it is stored correctly and readily retrieved. Patients should rehearse the information and skills verbally and mechanically with the health care provided so that he or she can assess whether the patient understands the information and can satisfactorily carry out the behaviors.

Beliefs

Related to knowledge and skills are beliefs about oneself, the self-care regimen, the health care provider, and the disease or problem. For example, Hartman and Becker (1978) found adherence to be associated with patients' perceptions of the probability of illness occurring as a result of nonadherence, the severity of these conditions should they occur, the value of following the prescribed regimen, and the barriers that interfere with adherence. The components of belief identified by Hartman and Becker are related to the Health Beliefs Model (e.g., Becker & Maiman, 1975). Although the components of the Health Beliefs Model have been widely investigated, they often account for relatively small amounts of variance (Haynes, Taylor, Snow, & Sackett, 1979). Unfortunately, evidence for the effectiveness of belief change approaches to behavior change is mixed (Cummings, Becker, Kirscht, & Levin, 1981; Haefner & Kirscht, 1970; Weisenberg, Kegeles, & Lund, 1980). These results suggest that modification of beliefs may be necessary to consider when trying to increase adherence; however, such changes may not be sufficient.

Beliefs in the effectiveness of self-care, however, will only be helpful when patients believe that they are competent to carry out the behaviors. Believing that one is incompetent may be associated with thoughts and feelings that prevent one from carrying out self-care behaviors (Bandura, 1977). The health care provider needs to pay attention both to patients' beliefs about the disease and the self-care regimen and the patients' beliefs about their own capabilities.

Motivation

Although knowledge and beliefs themselves will provide some
motivation, they are not sufficient to sustain behavior. Patients
need to be reinforced for carrying out self-care behaviors. Reinforcements can be self-managed, in which case patients attribute
performing the self-care behavior satisfactorily to their own
efforts. Reinforcement also can come from external sources such
as the family or health care provider. For significant others to
provide reinforcement, they also need to be knowledgeable about
self-care, and their beliefs must be consistent with those of the
patient. Thus, it is important for the health care provider to include family members in the education program. The issue of
family involvement and social support is more complex than
might at first be considered. We will return to discuss this topic
when we describe approaches to adherence enhancement later
in this chapter.

Failure to self-reinforce or to obtain external reinforcement
for self-care may result in a decline in carrying out self-care behaviors that were performed earlier during the course of the
disease. The patient must learn how to perceive each self-care
behavior as reinforcing. First, the patient needs to believe that
his or her actions are connected to the result, that is, results are
contingent on their own behaviors. Second, the patient needs to
interpret a positive result as reinforcing and a negative result as
a cue to examine his or her behavior and modify it. Interpreting
negative results as failures or punishments will most likely lead
to nonadherence rather than better adherence. For example, a
patient may think, "What's the use of trying?" or "I knew I
wouldn't be able to stay in good control," or "Nothing I do seems
to help." These thoughts and feelings occur frequently to patients
who try very hard to stick to the self-care program but are unable
to do so, or for whom adherence does not lead to improvement or
maintenance of health. In these patients, a sense of helplessness
and despair is quite common, and those feelings often contribute
to a lack of effort in trying to follow the regimen. On the other
hand, patients often do not interpret a positive result as a reinforcer but just a "matter of course." For example, some diabetic
patients do interpret a normal urine test as reinforcing but paradoxically view it in a maladaptive way. For example, patients

use the satisfactory results of the test as an indicator that they do not need to continue with the regimen as carefully since they are in good control.

Since it is likely that most, and perhaps all, patients—especially those who must continue complex and intrusive self-care programs for lengthy periods of time (e.g., diabetics, hypertensives, hemodialysis patients)—will fail to perform some behaviors at some time, the health care provider must consider what Marlatt and Gordon (1980) have called the "abstinence violation effect." That is, patients or people trying to maintain weight loss, smoking reduction, or reduced fluid intake view one "slip" as an indication of their lack of will power, incompetence, lack of control, or helplessness, and give up adhering despite the fact that they have been performing the appropriate behaviors for some time.

Action

Self-care includes a variety of behaviors that must be carried out in many different situations and often over a long period of time. The usual situation is the daily routine that the patient follows dealing with everyday problems and demands. Many of these behaviors may be time-consuming and aversive, and the patient has negative thoughts and feelings associated with them. The patient needs to deal with any thoughts or feelings that might inhibit carrying out self-care. The demands increase when the patient has to carry out the self-care behaviors in a problematic or atypical situation. The patient needs to feel confident that he or she knows what to do and is competent to handle unusual circumstances as they arise. We will consider how this may be accomplished later. Finally, the patient has to deal with the responses and attitudes of others with regard to his or her self-care behaviors.

In order to carry out these overt actions, patients need to attend to relevant internal cues, retrieve information from memory in the appropriate situation, and make discriminations, evaluations, and judgments. In short, patients must be able to discriminate the symptom, identify maladaptive thoughts or feelings, evaluate the seriousness of each, decide what action to take, and then follow through with the action.

Feedback

Since the components in self-care are interactive, of particular importance is the notion that actions provide feedback to knowledge and skills, beliefs, and motivation. Self-care is not static; changes occur over time as a result of the behaviors of the patient, health care provider, and significant others, and with the course of the disease. Successes in dealing with a problematic situation should be reinforcing and help the patient to feel more competent. On the other hand, failures to deal effectively may have negative consequences.

Feedback from any action requires that the patient interpret the experience accurately. Rather than automatically knowing how to interpret an action as a success or failure, patients may have to learn how to assess various situations. The patient needs to interpret successes and failures as cues for future actions. In terms of success, it is easy to understand how the patient will be encouraged to continue with the appropriate action; however, it is less clear how a failure should be interpreted so that it leads to proper self-care in the future. The reason for a failure can be anything—forgetting, unpredictable circumstances, laziness, or incomplete information. The patient needs to accept failure as only a temporary event, something that will occasionally occur but something that should not prevent subsequent self-care. Ideally, failure feedback should be viewed as a cue to reassess what has been done and to modify behaviors accordingly.

Adherence is a complex process. Factors at a number of levels influence whether a patient will carry out the self-care regimen. The inadequacies of traditional treatments may be a result of their failure to take into account individual patient differences in lifestyle; thoughts and feelings that accompany the disease and its treatment; internal processing of the information; beliefs; and motivations and external sources of reinforcement, such as family, friends, and the primary health care provider. In developing a self-care regimen, the health care provider should tailor the education program to meet the needs, problems, and concerns of the individual. Individualizing the self-care regimen, including consideration of the range of factors identified that can lead to nonadherence, is more likely to lead to effective and prolonged self-care by the patient.

ENHANCING ADHERENCE

One important virtue of the cognitive-behavioral perspective is that it suggests specific techniques that are likely to improve adherence to health care regimens. The cognitive-behavioral perspective places as much emphasis on the self-care enhancement process as it does on specific adherence enhancing techniques (Turk, Meichenbaum, & Genest, 1983).

A Collaborative Framework

An important characteristic of any attempt to increase long-term adherence is the creation of a collaborative framework in which both the patient and the health care provider share equally the responsibility of patient care (cf. Szasz & Hollander, 1956). Within such a framework, the patient and the health care provider work together to establish goals for self-care. Without the patient's cooperation, the most carefully designed and medically appropriate self-care regimen is likely to fail. The health care provider must be willing to compromise and perhaps relinquish some components of an idealized regimen that will not be followed for one that may be less ideal but that has some likelihood of being followed.

The role of the health care provider is to present relevant information, opinions, and options to the patient. The health care provider would like the patient to suggest what goals are important and what behaviors should be performed so that the patient comes to believe that he or she has contributed equally to the health care regimen. Ideally, the health care provider should attempt to orchestrate interactions so that the goals and behaviors suggested by the patient coincide with those that are most appropriate given the medical condition or health problem. It is important for the patient to announce explicitly his or her decision as to what goals he or she will work toward and what behaviors will be performed. Kanfer, Cox, Greiner, and Karoly (1974) and Janis and Mann (1977) report that such "public" announcement of intentions will have the effect of anchoring the person to the decision by anticipated social disapproval and self-disapproval and thus encourage adherence.

Care must be taken, however, to make sure that goals, or

subgoals, are not beyond the patient's capabilities. Early setbacks can lead to negative self-perceptions and lower feelings of self-efficacy. Thus, short-term goals that the patient can easily attain as well as moderate and long-term goals should be established. Moreover, the specific behaviors required to reach goals should be clearly presented. Setting goals that the patient will have minimal difficulty reaching, especially early on, is particularly important to enhance the patient's perception of self-competence.

In the colloaborative interchange, defensiveness should be minimized since the practitioner acts as a facilitator and advisor, and the patient develops a sense of internal commitment and personal causation in the process (Benfari et al., 1981; Turk et al., 1983). A number of recent studies have provided evidence to support the utility of the collaborative-negotiation model that is being advocated (e.g., Barofsky, 1978; Eisenthal, Emery, Lazare, & Udin, 1979; Roter, 1977; Schulman, 1979; Tracy, 1977). For example, Schulman (1979) studied the association of "active patient orientation" with learning blood pressure control by a group of hypertensive patients. An active patient orientation measure was designed to tap patients' perceptions of the extent to which they are "addressed as active participants involved in therapeutic planning and equipped to carry out self-care activities" (p. 278). Schulman (1979) found that patients who had higher scores on the patient orientation measure had greater blood pressure control, higher levels of adherence to prescribed health promoting activities, fewer medication side effects, and better understanding of treatment procedures.

A Problem-Solving Approach

Once a collaborative relationship is established, it becomes possible to adopt a problem-solving approach to the patient's self-care regimen. Problem-solving training includes a general problem-solving orientation as well as specific problem-solving skills. The problem-solving approach is geared toward helping the patient view the various self-care behaviors as tasks to be conducted. Atypical events or unusual situations that may interfere with adherence are viewed as problems to be resolved. Failures to adhere should also be approached as problems that can be solved.

The specific skills in problem-solving include the following: (a) acknowledging the presence of a problem, (b) clarifying the nature of the problem, (c) enumerating the possible solutions, (d) selecting a solution, and (e) testing it to determine whether the solution is adaptive (D'Zurilla & Goldfried, 1971). At first, the patient may need to focus on each stage of problem solving, but with practice the process should become automatic. An analogy that is helpful in explaining this to patients is that of learning to drive a standard transmission car (or learning to type). When someone first learns to drive, he or she is carefully attentive to each feature of driving—starting the motor, stepping on the clutch, shifting to first gear, accelerating, signaling, braking, stepping on the clutch, shifting again, and so forth. With repeated practice, each of these behaviors becomes automatic, receiving little direct attention from the driver.

Although problem-solving skills are necessary for adherence, they are not sufficient. Patients may be aware of all the components in problem solving but fail to act because they have negative thoughts or emotions associated with the problem that may interfere with problem resolution. Thus, failure to adhere can result from a deficiency in skills and knowledge or because something inhibits the performance of the appropriate behavior. If a patient fails to adhere to a therapeutic regimen, the health care provider should determine whether the patient has a deficiency in skills or knowledge or a deficiency in production of behaviors. When the patient acquires the needed skills to deal with the problems inherent in self-care and learns about the factors that inhibit production of the skills, he or she is more likely to carry out the self-care behaviors because of a sense of competence and, consequently, motivation is fostered.

The patient is encouraged to take responsibility for nonadherences as well as adherence. He or she should learn that failures should be viewed as problems that he or she should address and attempt to resolve in a manner similar to the health care provider. The questions that should come to the patient's mind when he or she becomes aware of not adhering or backsliding are "What factors contributed to my failure?" and "What can I do so that this doesn't happen again?" Problem solving is a mechanism by which the patients translate knowledge and information about their problem, treatment, and self-responsibility into behavior. The relative efficacy of problem-solving training has been demonstrated with several clinical populations (e.g., chronic pain patients, Acharya, Michaelson, & Erickson, 1978; cancer patients, Weisman, Worden, & Sobel, 1980; diabetic patients, Turk & Speers, 1981).

Although teaching the general steps in problem solving is important, the health care provider will likely achieve better results if he or she customizes the problem solving to each patient. When applying the approach with the individual patient, the health care provider should encourage the patient to be specific. For instance, a diabetic patient might say that he or she has a problem injecting insulin. This is a general statement of the patient's problem, but it lacks specificity. There are a host of possible causes of difficulty in injecting insulin such as "I'm afraid to give injections," "I do not get up at 7 a.m. every morning," "I do not want to inject into my stomach," or "I can not reach the area behind my arms to inject." Having the patient focus on the problem allows the health care provider to teach the patient in a manner directly relevant to him or her.

In the next stage, the health care provider and the patient generate possible solutions to each problem or task. Initially, the health care provider may spend more time explaining to the patient what to do, such as how to give an insulin injection; however, the patient can help the health care provider redefine the solution so that it is pertinent to his or her individual situation. The process of generating solutions will involve trial and error; solutions will have to be tried until the most adaptive ones are found for each patient.

An important point for the health care provider to keep in mind and to convey to patients is that of flexibility. Attempts to carry out many self-care behaviors, especially early on, are likely to result in some failures, setbacks, and plateaus in increased performance or goal attainment.

One chronic pain patient, seen by the first author, reported, in a rather despondent manner, that he had not performed the relaxation exercises that had been agreed upon. The patient in a dejected tone stated, "I knew I couldn't do it; it sounds good in practice, but I'm never good at sticking to things" (i.e., he has low self-efficacy). The patient was asked to describe what happened to interfere with the practice. He responded that he had relaxed for 10 minutes each night as agreed for three nights, but on the fourth night he did not, and he stopped doing the exercises completely. Additional probing revealed that the night he initially failed to adhere was related to the presence of company during the specified relaxation period. The next day when he realized that he had not performed the relaxation, he viewed this as confirmation of his inability to persevere (i.e., the abstinence violation effect). Surprisingly, this man never thought of the possibility of altering times of relaxation but seemed to stick rigidly to the schedule created. During the session, we worked with the patient on ways he could prevent similar problems in the future and how he could be flexible in modifying the treatment regimen with changing circumstances.

One of the major advantages to the problem-solving approach is that it actively involves the patient in the education process (Speers & Turk, 1982). By maintaining a continuous dialogue with the patient, the health care provider can assess many of the components of self-care adherence. Patients can tell the health care provider the following:

1. Their expectations, especially about what they hope to gain from the treatment regimen and health care providers.
2. Goals that can be negotiated and mutually agreed upon and ones that they feel will be carried out competently.
3. Beliefs that they have presently and ones that are lacking and will have to be instilled, such as the value of self-care in reducing long-term complications.
4. Problems in processing, storing, and retrieving information (for example, if a patient incorrectly answers a question about self-care, the health care provider will know that the information was not learned properly).
5. Cues in his or her environment that can be associated with self-care (since many skills are new, they will not occur automatically. One way to increase their occurrence is to have the patient connect the behavior, e.g., urine testing in diabetics, with a signal already present in his or her environment, such as brushing teeth in the morning).

6. Negative or interfering thoughts, emotions, or misconceptions.
7. Motivational deficits and problems (For example, the practitioner may need to encourage the patient to self-reinforce for good adherence).

Provision of Information

The provision of information is an important part of a cognitive-behavioral strategy to promote adherence. It is necessary to provide relevant information to the patient concerning his or her health problem. Although general medical knowledge does not appear to be associated with greater adherence (Haynes, 1976), a different kind of knowledge does appear to be related—namely, the extent to which the patient knows what behavior the regimen requires, and how and when to perform the behavior. Such knowledge is a necessary, but not sufficient, condition for following the regimen. A number of studies have indicated that this kind of information relates positively to adherence (Becker, Drachman, & Kirscht, 1972; Hulka, Cassel, & Kupper, 1976).

Instructions must be clear and precise and stated as simply as possible. The health care provider should make sure of the patient's understanding of the regimens before the patient leaves. This might be accomplished by questioning the patient as to when and how he or she might fulfill the regimens, what factors they can foresee that might interfere, and how these might be handled. To make sure the patient understands the specifics of the behaviors, it is helpful to have the patient tell the practitioner what it is, specifying what he or she is to do, and perhaps demonstrate the desired behavior.

One technique that we have found to be particularly helpful is role reversal. Patients who have been taught about self-care are asked to reverse roles, to pretend that they are the "expert" and they are trying to explain the self-care regimen to a novice patient (a role assumed by the health care provider). The role reversal technique serves three important functions. First, it enables the health care provider to learn about patients' understanding of the regimen, as well as their misconceptions and confusions. Second, it enables the patient to consolidate the knowledge and skills surrounding each behavior. Finally, the role reversal serves to allow the patient to generate arguments and explanations about self-care regimens that would be most likely to convince themselves of their merits. Social psychologists (e.g., Janis & King, 1954) have shown that when asked to role play, subjects will provide just the kinds of arguments that would be required to convince themselves of the merits of some perspective.

At the same time, it is necessary to provide a rationale for the treatment, both to clear up patients' misunderstandings about the regimen and to help patients become active participants in their own treatment. Kirscht and Rosenstock (1979), for example, report that hypertensive patients who were not sure of their treatment or of their condition were less likely to adhere to a regimen of prescribed drugs or dietary advice.

In addition to providing the information discussed, the health care provider must also assess the patient's ability to carry out the regimen (Speers & Turk, 1982). In complex regimens (for instance with diabetes, in which self-injection may be part of the treatment), the practitioner may have to model, or demonstrate, the correct procedure and have the patient practice it in the office.

Focusing on Beliefs: Cognitive Restructuring

In general, what people believe influences their achievement and maintenance of behavioral change, in this case adhering to a medical regimen. It is, therefore, important for the health care provider to attend to the beliefs of the patient and to try to encourage the patient to change beliefs that may undermine adherence. Perhaps the most persuasive arguments are those the patient generates for himself or herself. Thus, health care providers should try to have patients come to realize that their beliefs are maladaptive rather than simply telling them so. Using reflective responses and a perplexed demeanor may be helpful in carrying this out. For example, with one of our hypertensive patients, the following exchange occurred:

> P: Well, I've been feeling pretty good, so I stopped taking my pills and checking my blood pressure.

HCP: Oh, when you are feeling good, your blood pressure is low?

P: Yeah.

HCP: Have you noticed that your blood pressure goes up when you are not feeling good?

P: No, not really.

HCP: Then, I'm puzzled. It seems what you're saying is that how you are feeling doesn't really relate to the level of your blood pressure. Yet, you stopped checking your blood pressure because you have been feeling well.

P: I see what you mean. I can't really tell about my blood pressure without checking it every day.

In particular, the practitioner should attend to negative or maladaptive self-statements (e.g., "This medication schedule is too complicated. I'll never get it right"). These kinds of statements undermine the patient's perceived self-efficacy. To assess these cognitions, health care providers should elicit from patients their level of confidence regarding their ability to fulfill different parts of the regimen. If maladaptive cognitions are encountered, the health care provider must aid the patient in becoming aware of those thoughts, facilitate the collection of objective data to refute them, and encourage the production of adaptive self-statements that convey a realistic notion of the patient's self-efficacy. If proper rapport has been established and an objective or problem-solving approach to the treatment process has been adopted, then this type of cognitive change will come more easily to the patient.

Focusing on Behaviors: Contingency Contracting

Related to the idea of establishing and meeting goals in a collaborative framework is the practice of contingency contracting. This procedure involves a contract (often written) between the patient and the health care provider in which the patient agrees to abide by the contract by meeting goals in return for some reward (e.g., information, refund of a percent of treatment fees). Contingency contracting provides a systematized way for the health care provider to help in formulating realistic ways to achieve goals and to monitor any subsequent behavior (Kirscht & Rosenstock, 1979; Mahoney & Thoreson, 1974).

In some cases, contingency contracting may be an effective strategy. First, the process of developing the contract involves patients in the planning of their own regimen and thus gives them responsibility for its outcome. Second, the details of the regimen or prescription cannot be forgotten because they are written in the contract. Third, public commitment is elicited, helping to anchor the person to his or her decision. And fourth, the contract provides incentive value through the establishment of rewards for attainment of a self-established goal, thus making the personal accomplishment more salient.

In addition to specifically stating goals, expectancies, and reinforcements in a summary contract, we have found it helpful to use regular progress charts of goal attainment (cf. Fordyce, 1976). Patients keep charts of their performance of each self-care behavior. This serves as a constant reminder of the behaviors to be performed and provides continuous feedback about progress to both the participants and the health care provider. In this manner, problems and relapses are readily apparent and can be addressed before they become chronic, intractable problems that undermine adherence.

The use of such contracts has been found to be successful in fostering adherence for such problems as obesity (Dinoff, Rickard, & Colwick, 1972; Harris & Bruner, 1971), hypertension (Steckel & Swain, 1977), and chronic pain (Sternbach, 1974). A key part of the procedure used by Steckel and Swain was involvement of outpatients in the formal negotiation of an adherence contract, permitting the participants to choose adherence behaviors that they would perform during the contract's term and that would be rewarded if fulfilled, and then to assist in analyzing the process into manageable steps.

A "contract group," which also received patient education and standard medical attention, was compared with a group that received education plus standard care, and a standard care alone group. The major results of this study revealed that the patients in the contract group were all in good blood pressure control at a 15-month and a 30-month follow-up whereas the other two groups showed considerable fluctuation in blood pressure control. Furthermore, none of the patients in the contract group revealed any failures to adhere to the contract behaviors nor did any drop out of treatment. In contrast, 56 percent of the patients in the education plus standard care group and 28 percent of the patients in the standard care alone group dropped out of treatment.

In contrast to these generally positive results, a recent study reported by Cummings et al. (1980) revealed that behavioral contracts had only short-term adherence enhancement effects for a group of hemodialysis patients. The contract developed by Cummings et al. was similar to that employed by Steckel and Swain (1977), and consisted of (a) identifying a behavior or set of behaviors to be targeted for change in the contract; (b) negotiating with the patient a timetable for the accomplishment of the specified behaviors, how degree of accomplishment should be evaluated, what reward would be received for appropriate behavior, and when the patient would be rewarded; and (c) maintaining a record of each patient's progress. One possible explanation for the inconsistency in the results reported by Steckel and Swain (1977) and Cummings et al. relates to the complexity of the self-care regimen. The self-care regimen required of hemodialysis patients is quite a bit greater than that for hypertensives. Thus, the health care provider must be cautious in generalizing results from one population to another. In retrospect, it seems intuitively obvious that complex regimens require more than a behavioral contract to assure adherence.

Contingency contracting seems to be especially effective as an initial means of producing adherence behaviors and successes. A good strategy might be to gradually shift the emphasis from extrinsic to intrinsic rewards to sustain adherence over the long term. It is difficult for a health care professional to ensure the continuation of self-care behaviors that may not be intrinsically rewarding nor necessarily resulting in beneficial short-term efforts. Reinforcement must be transferred to the patient if adherence is to be maintained. The health care provider needs to assist the patient in recognizing the importance of adherence and to accept the responsibility for his or her own role in the self-care process (Haynes, Taylor, & Sackett, 1979). It is important to include concrete discussions of specific behaviors that are to be performed and how they are to be carried out in order to fulfill the contract and claim any reward (for an example of such a contract, see D'Andrea & Salovey, 1983).

An important caution about contingency contracting needs to be mentioned. There has been some debate about the long-term value of contingency contracting. We want to reiterate the cognitive-behavioral emphasis on collaboration between health care professionals and patients. The goals and self-care behaviors that have been noted should be negotiated and accepted by both parties. An important additional message is that the patient has some responsibility for failure but also for success. Thus, we are urging the health care provider to foster self-attributions of success by patients. In short, the health care provider can assist patients and teach them some things, but the performance of the behavior remains in the patients' control. Only patients can bring about appropriate behavior, and they should attribute both performance and lack of performance to their own efforts (Kopel & Arkowitz, 1975).

Social Support

Whenever possible, support (reinforcement, encouragement) should come from the health care provider. But he or she may also be in a position to arrange, or help the patient arrange, a support network away from the health care setting where the patient is the most vulnerable. Relatively little attention has been given to the role of social supports in adherence. In fact, the results of research on the effects of social support are somewhat mixed. For example, Hartman and Becker (1978) found that hemodialysis patients who reported fewer family problems and received more assistance from their spouses adhered better to a dietary regimen. Brownell, Heckerman, Westlake, Hayes, and Monti (1978) reported that partner support was associated with success in behavioral treatments for obesity. And, Caplan, Robinson, French, Coldwell, and Schinn (1976) found that hypertensive patients who were highly motivated to adhere and had a high degree of social support from their spouses achieved the highest levels of blood pressure control. On the other hand, Caplan et al. (1976) and Cummings et al. (1981) found that increasing social support had only short-term benefits on adherence. Moreover, Wilson and Brownell (1978) reported little benefit of including family members in the treatment of obesity and Cummings et al. (1981) found little association between support given by family members and adherence of hemodialysis patients.

The conflicting results regarding the benefits of family member inclusion in the treatment of obesity reported by Brownell and his colleagues (Brownell, Heckerman, Westlake, Haynes, & Monti, 1978; Wilson & Brownell, 1978) should sensitize health care providers to the point that support should not be confused with involvement. That is, simply bringing in family members or other "supportive people" does not guarantee that these people will be perceived by the patient as supportive. It is particularly important that more attention be given to the nature of the support rather than to its mere presence. As Stuart and Davis (1972) noted in studying eating patterns of obese women, "husbands are not only contributors to their wives' efforts to lose weight, but they may actually exert a negative influence." Family members may have good intentions and may try to be supportive, but they may do so inappropriately (for an extended review of this topic see Colletti & Brownell, 1982). What these data suggest is that involvement of family support may require a good deal of attention to teaching support people how to be of most benefit (Fordyce, 1976; Turk, Meichenbaum, & Genest, 1983).

Stress Inoculation and Relapse Prevention

Another kind of information that should be provided is directed specifically at preparing the patient for setbacks and relapse. Several studies have indicated that preparatory communications containing forewarnings about expected problems in adhering with realistic assurances that the patient can deal with such problems can function as stress inoculation to increase the patient's adherence to difficult decisions (Janis & Mann, 1977; Meichenbaum, 1977).

For example, although Caplan et al. (1976) could find no reasons for the lapse in adherence among the experimental groups, an examination of their procedure reveals no *active* attempt to prepare the patients for expectable setbacks or lack of progress.

What preparation that was provided consisted of discussion of possible reasons why people might stop adhering and possible ways to deal with those problems. It is possible that subjects in these groups were simply demoralized by setbacks because they were unable to cope with them and stopped adhering as a result.

The results of the studies on the role of information can be interpreted in terms of the information sources that affect a patient's self-efficacy. If a patient accepts a regimen without being aware of what it entails, and then finds it is more difficult than he or she at first believed, he or she may discontinue it. By providing full information and preparing the patient for possible difficulties, the patient should be less likely to blame himself or herself for his or her setback and more likely to see it as a problem that can be solved.

According to Meichenbaum (1977), however, merely warning a patient of what may happen may not be sufficient to ward off failures, or perceived failures, in adherence. One feature of a stress inoculation program that might be added has been suggested by Janis and Rodin (1979). They point out that forewarnings designed to prevent backsliding are more likely to be effective if the person has committed himself to his decision and that commitment is enhanced by exposure to a minor challenge that can be easily overcome by the patient. Janis and Rodin suggest that health care providers might present such a mild challenge themselves after the person has announced his decision to adhere, by calling attention to unpleasant consequences of the treatment program. By allowing the patient an opportunity to overcome a small challenge of this sort, the patient makes a personal accomplishment that bolsters self-efficacy.

It is uncertain whether such programs can be very effective in combatting real-life setbacks or lack of progress. This is especially problematic in cases like hypertension in which good adherence to treatment produces few noticeable changes. As a result of their study of alcoholics, Chaney et al. (1978) assert that approaches that use *only* verbal persuasion or supportive social groups do not assist the client in reevaluating expectations of personal efficacy. This is consistent with Bandura's (1977) assertion that *enactive mastery* produces the highest, strongest, and most generalized increases in coping efficacy.

What is being argued for, then, is an approach that allows the patient to anticipate problems and to actively rehearse coping strategies to deal with those problems. Meichenbaum and Turk (1976) have developed a stress inoculation program that involves three main steps that can be considered guidelines for effective inoculation programs: (1) provide the patient with a conceptual framework of the stress reaction and motivate him or her to acquire coping skills with which to counter the stress, (2) teach the patient specific coping skills to deal with stressful events and have the patient rehearse those skills, and (3) have the patient practice and apply the coping skills to specific, predictable stressful situations and then generalize them to unplanned circumstances. This can be done by means of role playing in imagined stressful situations or by actual exposure to real-life stresses. Ideally, self-statements made during such a stress inoculation should be directed toward anticipating coping behaviors or reconceptualizing situations into nonthreatening terms (Girodo, 1977).

Chaney et al. (1978) attempted to modify efficacy expectation in alcoholics through corrective experience and skills training (following Meichenbaum & Turk, 1976). The study compared three groups of alcoholics in a controlled-drinking program. The experimental group received a program of skill training that include modeling, role playing, coaching techniques to work through the problem-solving steps of problem definition and formulation, generation of alternatives, and decision making, and then rehearsing optimal alternatives. A discussion-only group talked about the same situations that the experimental group practiced solving but did not use modeling, role playing, or coaching. A second control group received no additional training beyond the regular treatment regimen.

The results indicated that during the posttreatment year, the drinking behavior of the skills training group and the control groups (discussion-only and regular medical treatment only) significantly diverged as measured by days intoxicated, quantity of alcohol consumed, and duration of drinking periods. These results show promise for a program of inoculation against backsliding in adherence situations. A relapse prevention program (e.g., Chaney et al., 1978; Turk et al., 1983) may be especially promising because it concentrates on identifying real high-risk situations and actively rehearsing ways to cope with them.

Since it is unlikely that health care professionals can anticipate all high-risk situations, it may be important to reinforce the
general problem-solving orientation noted earlier by having patients acknowledge that unforseen problems will likely occur but
that the patient is competent to deal with these as they arise. One
procedure that can assist in generating possible problem situations
is called "outcome psychodrama" (Janis & Mann, 1977). Outcome psychodrama is a kind of role playing in which the patient
is asked to play the role of himself at some moment in time after
he has made his decision to adhere. Additionally, the health care
provider may suggest specific situations, or best-case and worst-
case scenarios, for the patient to imagine. A typical psychodrama
might have the patient going through the events of an average
work day, or weekend day, and imagine specific situations and
his reactions to the situations. This can be an effective method for
generating the kinds of problem situations that might be stressful
and demoralizing but that could be anticipated.

SUMMARY

The cognitive-behavioral approach to enhancement of adherence
conceptualizes the process as consisting of seven phases with a
number of primary goals for each phase. We have summarized
these phases and goals in Table 4.1; however, it is important to
note that the phases are not mutually exclusive or rigid steps
existing in a nonoverlapping sequence. Although some phases
stand in temporal relation to others, other phases occur simultaneously. The *process* should be viewed as dynamic and not
necessarily lockstep. We present these stages separately and
hierarchically simply for clarity. In many ways, these phases
and goals are analogous to the cognitive-behavioral perspective
on counseling and psychotherapy (cf. Kanfer & Grimm, 1980;
Turk et al., 1983).

We have described several techniques to enhancing patient
adherence (e.g., social support, contingency contracting, stress
inoculation, cognitive restructuring); however, we are less concerned about the specifics of techniques than the general perspective offered. From a cognitive-behavioral perspective, no durable
change is expected unless three general conditions are met: (1) the

TABLE 4.1*   Phases of Adherence

Phase	Primary Goals
Role structuring and creating a collaborative relationship	Forming of a working relationship Establishing motivation Creating an expectancy of success Fostering a sense of active patient participation
Creating commitment for self-care	Motivate patient to consider positive consequences of self-care Activate patient toward change Combat sense of passivity and helplessness
Cognitive-functional analysis	Identify functional relationships among thoughts, feelings, and behaviors Clarify misconceptions Motivate toward specific goals Problem-solving orientation
Negotiating self-care regimen	Seek agreement on target behaviors Establish priorities for self-care Accept responsibility for performing self-care progress
Self-care execution and motivation maintenance	Provide relevant information Skills training Assess effects of self-care behavior Evaluate and, if necessary, enhance motivation to change and adhere to self-care requirements
Monitoring and evaluating self-care	Assess performance of self-care behaviors Assess use of problem-solving orientation Assess use of general coping skills Modify self-care behaviors, if necessary
Generalization and maintenance	Evaluate and, if necessary, enhance motivation to change and adhere to self-care requirements Relapse prevention

*Adapted from Kanfer and Grimm, 1980.

patient accepts (or is led to accept) the therapeutic objectives because of his or her expected value for them rather than their worth to the health care provider, (2) the patient attributes ultimate success or failure to his or her own behavior, and (3) the patient believes he or she is competent to carry out the self-care regimen (i.e., develops high self-efficacy). There are any number of ways to try and bring these conditions about (e.g., Cormier & Cormier 1979; Kanfer & Goldstein, 1975; Kendall & Hollon,

1979), and at present there are no definitive techniques. Rather, we would encourage creative development and utilization of innovative approaches as long as they are designed to foster patient motivation, responsibility, and perceived competence.

REFERENCES

Acharya, A., Michaelson, M. A., & Erickson, D. L. *Use of a problem-solving approach in the treatment of chronic pain.* Paper presented at the 2nd World Congress on Pain, Montreal, Canada, August, 1978.

Bandura, A. Self-efficacy: Toward a unified theory of behavioral change. *Psychological Review, 84,* 191–215, 1977.

Bandura, A. The self system in reciprocal determinism. *American Psychologist, 33,* 344–358, 1978.

Barofsky, I. Compliance, adherence and the therapeutic alliance: Steps in the development of self-care. *Social Science and Medicine, 12,* 369–376, 1978.

Becker, M. H., Drachman, R., Kirscht, R. H., & Kirscht, D. P. Predicting mothers' compliance with pediatric medical regimens. *Journal of Pediatrics, 81,* 843–854, 1972.

Becker, M. H., & Maiman, L. A. Sociobehavioral determinants of compliance with health and medical recommendations. *Medical Care, 13,* 10–24, 1975.

Benfari, R. C., Eaker, E., & Stoll, J. G. Behavioral interventions and compliance to treatment regimes. *Annual Review of Public Health, 2,* 431–465, 1981.

Brownell, K. D., Heckerman, C. L., Westlake, R. J., Hayes, S. C., & Monti, P. M. The effect of couples training and partner cooperativeness in behavioral treatment of obesity. *Behavior Research and Therapy, 16,* 323–333, 1978.

Caplan, R., Robinson, E. A. R., French, J. R. P., Jr., Caldwell, J. R., & Schinn, M. *Adhering to medical regimens.* Ann Arbor: Institute for Social Research, 1976.

Cassata, D. M. Health communication theory and research: An overview of the communication specialist interface. In D. Nimmo (Ed.), *Communication yearbook II.* New York: ICA, 1978.

Chaney, E., O'Leary, M., & Marlatt, G. A. Skill training with alcoholics. *Journal of Consulting and Clinical Psychology, 46,* 1092–1104, 1978.

Colletti, G., & Brownell, K. D. The physical and emotional benefits of social support-application to obesity, smoking, and alcoholism. In M. Hersen, R. M. Eisler, & P. M. Miller (Eds.), *Progress in behavior modification.* Vol. 13. New York: Academic Press, 1982.

Cormier, W. H., & Cormier, L. S. *Interviewing strategies for helpers: A guide to assessment, treatment, and evaluation.* Monterey, CA: Brooks/Cole, 1979.

Cummings, K. M., Becker, M. H., Kirscht, J. P., & Levin, N. W. Psychosocial factors affecting adherence to medical regimens in a group of hemodialysis patients. *Medical Care, 20,* 567–580, 1982.

D'Andrea, V. J., & Salovey, P. *Peer counseling: Skills and perspectives.* Palo Alto, CA: Science and Behavior Books, 1983.

Dinoff, M., Rickard, N. C., & Colwick, J. Weight reduction through successive contracts. *American Journal of Orthopsychiatry, 42,* 110–113, 1972.

DiMatteo, M. R., & DiNicola, D. D. *Achieving patient compliance.* New York: Pergamon, 1982.

Dunbar, J. Adhering to medical advice: A review. *International Journal of Mental Health, 9,* 70–87, 1980.

Dunbar, J., & Stunkard, A. Adherence to diet and drug regimen. In R. Levy, B. Rifkind, & N. Ernst (Eds.), *Nutrition, lipids, and coronary heart disease.* New York: Raven Press, 1979.

D'Zurilla, T. J., & Goldfried, M. R. Problem solving and behavior modification. *Journal of Abnormal Psychology, 78,* 107–126, 1971.

Eisenthal, S., Emery, R., Lazare, A., & Udin, H. 'Adherence' and the negotiated approach to patienthood. *Archives of General Psychiatry, 36,* 393–398, 1979.

Epstein, L. H., & Cluss, P. A. A behavioral medicine perspective on adherence to long-term medical regimens. *Journal of Consulting and Clinical Psychology, 50,* 950–971, 1982.

Fordyce, W. E. *Behavioral methods for chronic pain and illness.* St. Louis: C. V. Mosby, 1976.

Girodo, M. Self-talk: Mechanisms in anxiety and stress management. In C. D. Spielberger & I. G. Sarason (Eds.), *Stress and anxiety.* Vol 4. Washington, DC: Hemisphere, 1977.

Haefner, D. P., & Kirscht, J. P. Motivational and behavioral effects of modifying health beliefs. *Public Health Reports, 55,* 478–484, 1970.

Harris, M. B., & Bruner, C. G. A comparison of self-control and a contract procedure for weight control. *Behavior Research and Therapy, 9,* 347–354, 1971.

Hartman, P. E., & Becker, M. H. Noncompliance with prescribed regimen among chronic hemodialysis patients: A method of prediction and educational diagnosis. *Dialysis and Transplantation, 7,* 978–989, 1978.

Haynes, R. B. A critical review of the "determinants" of patient compliance with therapeutic regimens. In D. L. Sackett & R. B. Haynes (Eds.), *Compliance with therapeutic regimens.* Baltimore, MD: Johns Hopkins University Press, 1976.

Haynes, R. B., Taylor, D. W., & Sackett, D. L. *Compliance in health care.* Baltimore, MD: Johns Hopkins University Press, 1979.

Haynes, R. B., Taylor, D. W., Snow, J. C., & Sackett, D. L. Annotated and indexed bibliography on compliance with therapeutic and preventive regimens. In R. B. Haynes, D. W. Taylor, & P. L. Sackett (Eds.), *Compliance in health care.* Baltimore, MD: Johns Hopkins University Press, 1979.

Hochbaum, G. M. Why do people seek diagnostic x-rays? *Public Health Reports, 71,* 377–380, 1956.

Hulka, B. S., Cassel, J. C., & Kupper, L. L. Disparities between medications prescribed and consumed among chronic disease patients. In L. Lasagna (Ed.), *Patient compliance.* Mt. Kisco, NY: Futura, 1976.

Janis, I. L., & King, B. The influence of role-playing on opinion change. *Journal of Abnormal and Social Psychology, 49,* 211–218, 1954.

Janis, I. L., & Mann, L. *Decision making.* New York: Free Press, 1977.

Janis, I. L., & Rodin, J. Attribution, control and decision making: Social psychology and health care. In G. Stone, F. Cohen, & N. Adler (Eds.), *Health psychology.* San Francisco: Jossey-Bass, 1979.

Kanfer, F. H., Cox, L. E., Greiner, J. M., & Karoly, P. Contracts, demand characteristics, and self-control. *Journal of Personality and Social Psychology, 30,* 605–619, 1974.

Kanfer, F. H., & Goldstein, A. P. (Eds.), *Helping people change.* New York: Pergamon Press, 1975.

Kanfer, F. H., & Grimm, L. G. Managing clinical change: A process model of therapy. *Behavior Modification, 1,* 419–444, 1980.

Kendall, P. C., & Hollon, S. D. (Eds.), *Cognitive-behavioral interventions: Theory, research, and procedures.* New York: Academic Press, 1979.

Kirscht, J. P., Kirscht, J. L., & Rosenstock, I. M. A test of interventions to increase adherence to hypertensive medical regimens. *Health Education Quarterly, 8,* 261–272, 1981.

Kirscht, J. P., & Rosenstock, I. Patients' problems in following recommendations or health experts. In G. Stone, F. Cohen, & N. Adler (Eds.), *Health psychology.* San Francisco: Jossey-Bass, 1979.

Kopel, S., & Arkowitz, H. The role of attribution and self-perception in behavior change: Implications for behavior therapy. *Genetic Psychology Monographs, 92,* 175–212, 1975.

Ley, P. Memory for medical information. *British Journal of Social and Clinical Psychology, 18,* 245–258, 1979.

Mahoney, M. J., & Mahoney, K. *Permanent weight control.* New York: W. W. Norton, 1976.

Mahoney, M. J., & Thoreson, C. E. *Self-control: Power to the person.* Monterey, CA: Brooks/Cole, 1974.

Marlatt, G. A., & Gordon, J. R. Determinants of relapse: Implications for the maintenance of behavior change. In P. O. Davidson & S. M. Davidson (Eds.), *Behavioral medicine: Changing health life styles.* New York: Brunner/Mazel, 1980.

Meichenbaum, D. H. *Cognitive-behavior modification: An integrative approach.* New York: Plenum, 1977.

Meichenbaum, D. H., & Turk, D. C. The cognitive-behavioral management of anxiety, anger, and pain. In P. O. Davidson (Ed.), *The behavioral management of anxiety, depression and pain.* New York: Brunner/Mazel, 1976.

Meichenbaum, D. H., & Turk, C. C. Stress, coping, and disease: A cognitive behavioral perspective. In R. W. J. Neufeld (Ed.), *Psychological stress and psychopathology.* New York: McGraw-Hill, 1982.

Richmond, J. *Healthy people; The Surgeon General's report on health promotion and disease prevention* (U.S. Department of Health, Education & Welfare (PHS) Publication No. 79–55071). Washington, DC: U.S. Government Printing Office, 1979.

Roter, D. L. Patient participation in the patient-provider interaction: The effects of patient question asking on the quality of interaction, satisfaction and compliance. *Health Education Monographs, 5,* 281–319, 1977.

Sackett, D. L., & Haynes, R. B. (Eds.), *Compliance with therapeutic regimens*. Baltimore, MD: Johns Hopkins University Press, 1976.

Schulman, B. A. Active patient orientation and outcomes in hypertensive treatment: Application of a socio-organizational perspective. *Medical Care, 17,* 267–280, 1979.

Speers, M. A., & Turk, D. C. Diabetes self-care: Knowledge, beliefs, motivation and action. *Patient Counselling and Health Education, 4,* 144–149, 1982.

Steckel, S., & Swain, M. The use of written contracts to increase adherence. *Hospitals, 51,* 81–84, 1977.

Sternbach, R. A. *Pain patients: Traits and treatment.* New York: Academic Press, 1974.

Stuart, R. B., & Davis, B. *Slim chance in a fat world: Behavioral control of obesity.* Champaign, IL: Research Press, 1972.

Szasz, T. S., & Hollander, M. H. A contribution to the philosophy of medicine. The basic models of the doctor-patient relationship. *Archives of Internal Medicine, 97,* 585–592, 1956.

Tracy, J. Impact of intake procedures upon client attrition in a community mental health center. *Journal of Consulting and Clinical Psychology, 45,* 192–196, 1977.

Turk, D. C., Meichenbaum, D. H., & Genest, M. *Pain and behavioral medicine: A cognitive-behavioral perspective.* New York: Guilford Press, 1983.

Turk, D. C., & Salovey, P. *Cognitive structures, cognitive processes, and cognitive-behavior modification: II. Clinical interference.* Manuscript submitted for publication, 1983.

Turk, D. C., & Speers, M. A. *Enhancing adherence to diabetic self-care regimens.* Paper presented at the 15th annual convention of the Association for the Advancement of Behavior Therapy, Toronto, November 1981.

Turk, D. C., & Speers, M. A. Cognitive schemata and cognitive processes in cognitive-behavioral interventions: Going beyond the information given. In P. C. Kendall (Ed.), *Advances in cognitive-behavioral research and therapy.* Vol. 2. New York: Academic Press, 1983.

Weisenberg, M., Kegeles, S. S., & Lund, A. K. Children's health beliefs and acceptance of a dental preventive activity. *Journal of Health and Social Behavior, 21,* 59–74, 1980.

Weisman, A. D., Worden, J. W., & Sobel, H. J. *Psychosocial screening and intervention with cancer patients: Research report.* Cambridge, MA: Shea Bros., 1980.

Wilson, G. T., & Brownell, K. D. Behavior therapy for obesity: Including family members in the treatment process. *Behavior Therapy, 9,* 943–945, 1978.

5

Compliance and the Quality of Survival

Alexis M. Nehemkis
Kenneth E. Gerber

In introducing the ideas of this book, we have said that one of us has thought intensively about end-stage renal disease patients, while the other has, for many years, pondered the psychological problems indigenous to "the cancer ward."

The experience of the chronic hemodialysis patient uniquely illustrates the philosophical and clinical complexity of compliance in chronic illness. Numerous articles beamed at a variety of psychosocial, medical, and nursing audiences have focused on personality and situational correlates of compliance to the dialysis regimen (Abram, 1974; Armstrong, 1978; Blodgett, 1981; Kaplan De-Nour & Czaczkes, 1972).

This literature makes clear that noncompliance colors every aspect of dialysis treatment. Indeed, as we stated in Chapter 1, most psychologists' responsibilities on the dialysis unit can be reduced to the issue of enhancing patients' compliance to their medical regimen.

The opposite is true of advanced cancer patients in whom the incidence of noncompliance to their likewise demanding treatment program is negligible. In this chapter we wish to explore these tandem questions about the patient populations of special interest to each of us.

Why is the multidimensional, configural nature of the compliance problem repetitive in the management of patients on a dialysis unit? And why is the problem a nonissue on the cancer ward? In each instance the behavior of these very different patient groups raises a number of important philosophical and clinical issues which we address in this chapter.

CHRONIC HEMODIALYSIS

The experience of the chronic hemodialysis patient uniquely illustrates the philosophical and clinical complexity of compliance in chronic illness. Numerous articles (Abram, 1974; Armstrong, 1978; Blodgett, 1981; Kaplan De-Nour & Czaczkes, 1972) addressed to a variety of psychosocial, medical, and nursing disciplines have focused on personality and situational correlates of compliance to the dialysis regimen. The first part of this chapter will provide a thorough review of the issue of compliance in this patient population leading to a broader view of the dilemma that faces patient and staff who are concerned with adherence to the dialysis regimen. In the second part we shall consider a different patient population—the population of advanced cancer patients—in which, by contrast, the incidence of noncompliance is negligible, but whose behavior, like that of their seriously ill counterparts on dialysis, raises a number of important philosophical and clinical issues.

The Plight of the Dialysis Patient

Chronic renal failure until recently spelled certain, relatively rapid death. The inability of the body to purge itself of poisonous urea, the by-product of protein metabolism, leads to the condition of uremia. Uremia is characterized by dizziness, nausea, vomiting, headache, elevated blood pressure and, eventually, coma leading to death. Dialysis, as an extracorporeal method of voiding toxins such as urea, was first used in experimental animal work early in this century. The first human use of dialysis was performed in 1943, by W. J. Kolff, a Dutch physician. In 1960, the first prolonged intermittent hemodialysis was reported. By the late 1960s, the procedure was available on a larger scale but was exceedingly expensive and physically stressful when performed on a chronic basis. It was offered only to a select few, chosen anonymously by a panel of medical and lay persons. In 1972, Medicare payments for hemodialysis were approved and treatment was offered on a large scale. Fifty thousand patients are now on maintenance dialysis in the United States. The treatment is unusual in that it offers no cure but simply maintains life. Patients still experience significant metabolic abnormalities as dialysis is a very imperfect procedure. Complications of the disease and treatment are multiple and complex.

Dialysis patients participate in an exceptionally demanding treatment regimen. Although treatment session time has decreased, patients still need three four-hour treatments per week. Transportation and waiting time increase the total hours to five to eight hours every other day. In short, patients spend three days every week involved in dialysis. Other medical tests and procedures are common and may fill up the remaining free time. Patients typically report feeling "washed out" after each dialysis as well as feeling tired, lethargic (i.e. uremic) prior to the run. An outline of the dialysis patient's week shows a "see-saw" effect of feeling poorly, then dialyzing, and feeling tired afterward, followed by a good day and then the cycle beginning again. The day-to-day life of a dialysis patient is characterized by a stressful routine within which there is never any option to delay or cancel a treatment. Each treatment is critical to bringing the body back into a state approaching metabolic equilibrium.

Examples abound of physical complications of chronic renal failure and the resulting dialysis treatment and occur in most patients who undergo chronic dialysis. They include the following, depending on the particular individual medical situation: peripheral neuropathy, blood glucose aberration, lethargy, sleep reversal irritability, confusion, headaches, nausea, blood pressure abnormalities, neuronal loss, bone disease, and neurological changes including metabolic encephalopathy, dialysis dementia, anemia, pericardial disease, and cardiomegaly. Patients are at high risk for hepatitis and duodenal ulcers. Low red blood cell production as measured by hematocrit level leads to chronic levels of weakness. All of the above complications of chronic renal failure and hemodialysis are magnified if certain other diseases underlie the renal failure.

Each dialysis encounter is a risk. Patients may experience painful muscle cramps, decreasing blood pressure ("crashing"), nausea, and vomiting. Needles may have to be stuck into the arm numerous times to ensure proper blood flow. Most patients have witnessed a fellow dialysand experience a myocardial infarction while undergoing the cardiovascularly stressful procedure. Patients are attached to a machine and remain helpless while their peer is "worked on" by the medical team. Each run is experienced as being very slow and monotonous. Patients may report the eerie sensation of feeling blood being pumped out of their body. Individuals are severely restricted in protein and potassium intake. Potassium is not only dangerous for a patient, but its ingestion must be monitored with the utmost precision. For minute changes in potassium—high levels of which are found in many common foods—may trigger deadly cardiac arrythmias. Fluid intake must be severely restricted, particularly if the patient is anuric. Patients must ingest large quantities of medication, including vitamins, phosphate binders, antihypertensives, and folic acid, often exceeding 50 pills per day. Food restriction becomes a critical issue for patients and family. Patients are known to dream about forbidden food and to identify food restriction as a major source of social/ domestic stress. Diabetes, a leading cause of chronic renal failure, demands an even more stringent diet, with added physical complications, including retinopathy and restricted peripheral blood flow. Such added physical problems severely affect patients' psychological functioning. Social areas are also affected. Patients are limited in making any type of spontaneous travel plans. Sessions cannot be missed, no matter how the person is feeling or whatever home or work demands are. Vocational demands are difficult to meet both because of physical condition and time pressures. Patients who make their living in physically demanding occupations are especially vulnerable to losing their livelihood. The dialysis patient's life is experienced as surviving on a slim margin between living and dying.

In the last few years, a greater promise has been offered by continuous ambulatory peritoneal dialysis (CAPD), with its more liberal dietary restrictions, as an alternative to hemodialysis. Patients also enjoy greater freedom with this method as it is administered by the patient himself, outside the hospital. CAPD consists of infusing a dialysate solution into the peritoneal cavity which, through an osmotic process, washes out waste product fluid normally eliminated in the urine. Although no needles are used and the patient needn't come into the clinic for the treatment, the procedure is very time-consuming, usually done four times per day, a total of, perhaps, 25 hours per week. Extreme cleanliness is a great necessity. CAPD is not as stressful on the body as hemodialysis, but it does not eliminate many of the complications of chronic renal disease documented above. Patients chosen for CAPD treatment clearly must show a high degree of self-reliance. It is unclear, however, what types of patients are the most compliant with the procedure's many demands (Burton et al., 1983). Even though CAPD may eliminate some of the compliance requirements of hemodialysis, it appears to substitute other compliance demands if only because the patient conducts the treatment with minimal supervision. CAPD is a relatively new procedure which has generated considerable optimism. It is, however, becoming increasingly clear that this technique has many of the psychological complications of hemodialysis. For example, Benjamin (1983) has written of his own experience on CAPD, outliving the difficulties of the procedure and, at least for him, its overall unpleasantness. CAPD, a seemingly promising option for the chronic renal failure patient, cannot be said to totally eliminate the problems of dialysis so far discussed.

The Problem of Compliance

Compliance is an obvious issue in a number of areas previously described: medication, fluid, protein, potassium restriction, and punctuality in coming to treatment. In addition, dialysis unit staff (Gerber, 1984) have identified other factors defining compliance. These include patients' willingness to do some self-care activities (e.g., setting up prep trays), being friendly toward staff, and not complaining about unit care. Early research with dialysis patients identified noncompliance as a serious problem. Kaplan De-Nour and Czaczkes (1972) determined that only 50 percent of patients they studied were, overall, compliant with medical regimen. Other studies place the range of noncompliance between 5 and 92 percent. Rates vary according to the measurement technique. For example, objective measures of compliance such as blood chemistries yield higher noncompliance rates than do patient self-report measures. In the exercise of compliance, patients exhibit a complex set of behaviors. Although typically compliance is defined in general terms, it is critical to define the specific component behaviors. For example, Kaplan De-Nour and Czaczkes (1976) have concluded that patients can be compliant in one area and noncompliant in another. Thousands of medical, psychological, and nursing studies have tried to identify the factors predicting positive adjustment of a patient to the rigorous life previously described. Critical psychosocial issues for the patient include coming to terms with the dependence on a machine for survival, changed body image, dietary and travel restrictions, feeling poorly much of the time, family stresses related to dialysis, problems in sexual performance, loss of group membership, and vocational restrictions. Low frustration tolerance and high levels of acting-out are common problems. Depression is a common symptom. Psychological approaches for increasing compliance have often included behavioral methods, such as contracting, modeling, cueing, or more traditional methods, such as group therapy.

"The Too-Long Life"

The dilemma of the dialysis patient is clearly more complex than simply emitting certain behaviors that define compliance. We believe it is best to view the dialysis patient's life circumstance as signifying a path of crisis. Becoming a dialysis patient involves being suddenly removed from the ordinary context of one's life. Abram (1974) has observed that the patient attempts to live the "too-long life"—a sense of life going on longer than it was meant to. In a much quoted paper, Alexander (1976) asserts that the patient on dialysis enters a perfect double-bind relationship with family and staff. Patients are encourage to be independent and act "well"; however, the essence of dialysis is dependence on others to live and to be ill. Independent behavior is thus both encouraged and denied. Zaner (1980), a philosopher who comments on the dillemmas of the dialysis patient, identifies the patient's continuous encounter with dying and death as establishing the critical background to his subjective experience. The critical issue for the dialysis patient is nothing less than a moral dilemma. The staff request of the patient that he have courage and trust is not an issue amenable to technique, but rather demands that we address the fundamental notions of "what is a life worth living?" The essence of chronic illness is the lack of cure. Thus, dependence, limitations, and "chronic dying" all characterize the condition. The everyday sense of life, "the taken-for-grantedness" that colors most lives, is severely shaken by the condition. We can no longer expect that patients will choose to do the right thing, i.e., comply the way most of us say we would behave if in the same situation. Patients must become chronically dependent on strangers whom they may neither like nor trust. Trust, however, is complicated by the fact that dialysis is known to be imperfect, fraught with medical and technical complications. The patient's course is inexorably downward. The courage we ask of such patients must be tempered by the knowledge of their phenomenological experience. Unlike the experience of many terminally ill patients who know their suffering will soon cease, dialysis patients do not experience an intensification of living, a sharpening of the senses, or a heightened appreciation of life. Theirs is the too-long life, in the evocative phrase of Unamuno. Each dialysis session which rescues the patient from certain death ironically reminds him of his own mortality. Patients experience a great sense of injustice, an injustice that has no end.

Unique Dilemmas of Dialysis: The Themes of Existentialism

Yalom (1980) has written of the relevance of the theoretical principles of existentialism to understanding the experience of the medical patient. To be sure, the four principles he identifies must be considered when trying to understand the experience of being a dialysis patient. The dialysis patient's sense of isolation from others, his constant awareness of being near death, the need to feel a purpose in his very special life circumstances, and the notion of responsibility for his life (i.e., for becoming ill and for living with the illness) are all fundamental issues for the chronic renal failure patient kept alive by a machine. To Yalom, such principles are critical to all human beings but are acutely experienced in the seriously ill patient. Working in the clinical setting with dialysis patients quickly dispels any notion that such concerns are either overly abstract, superfluous, or irrelevant to psychological intervention. Indeed, our experience indicates that noncompliance in this patient group—with the exception of successful informational interventions for helping a new patient to learn his diet—can only be understood and treated with a thorough appreciation of how the patient perceives these basic concepts within his own life. In the dialysis population these concepts often translate into ambivalence toward routine dialysis treatment and, thus, toward living. Such ambivalence ensures a continuous level of noncompliance, as motivation to "be well" fluctuates from day to day. Ambivalence toward complying is further intensified by the patient's sense of isolation from those around him who do not experience life on dialysis. We believe these concepts must be addressed with dialysis patients in order to understand patient behavior. Intervention focused only on overt behavior will, in most cases, produce insignificant, temporary behavior change. Yalom, in summarizing the essence of addressing existential concepts in psychotherapy, emphasizes the phenomenological approach. Here, the therapist attempts to enter the world of the patient without "standardized instruments and presuppositions" (Yalom, 1980, p. 25). Therapy does not revolve around comparing the patient to normative standards (e.g., compliant or noncompliant) but rather explores the patient's dealing with the basic existential themes, (i.e., death, freedom, isolation, meaning of life). These core existential concerns, as noted above, seem particularly relevant to chronically ill dialysis patients.

Patient Compliance as a Staff Problem

What determines the designation of a patient as either compliant or noncompliant? Kaplan De-Nour, a psychiatrist who pioneered the psychological study of the dialysis patient, writes convincingly that noncompliance is a staff, and not a patient, problem. Based on her recent work (Kaplan De-Nour, 1982), it can be said that the compliance issue reflects a complex and unspoken lack of agreement between staff and patients regarding what is the appropriate "quality of life" on the dialysis machine. (Chapter 8 is devoted in its entirety to this issue). Research has indicated that highly skilled dialysis nurses often project unrealistic expectations on patients resulting in both staff and patient frustration and depressions. Staff disillusionment is well documented and is related to the frustration of attempting to treat patients whose condition will never improve and who do not take perfect care of themselves. One of the clearest illustrations of this phenomenon is seen in the case of B.G., a 60-year-old Mexican-American patient with malignant hypertension leading to chronic renal failure. He chronically suffered from an ulcer. He demanded blood transfusions whenever his hematocrit fell to 19 or 20, stating that this condition produced headaches, tinnitus, and nervousness. Staff refused to allow this because regular bimonthly transfusions would eventually shut down all natural red blood cell production, leaving the patient—at some distant point in the future—totally dependent on transfusions. Arguments predictably ensued every few months as the patient reported the set of symptoms that demanded transfusion. When the patient was interviewed, it became apparent that this otherwise cooperative patient experienced a very different set of priorities than did staff. He spoke of his anger at staff for holding back a treatment that would make his daily life tolerable. His concern for the distant future was minimal. His symptoms were so aversive that the present was all that mattered. B.G. clearly understood the facts about hematocrit, blood transfusions, and their relationship to renal failure. He expressed himself succinctly: "I do the best I can with dialysis. If I have to live with it, I will, but not this way. I don't want to live feeling this way." Staff expressed consternation that he would make such a choice. Once B.G. was labeled by staff as "difficult," the characterization of "noncompliant" was not far behind. Henceforth, his behavior was more closely scrutinized for added evidence of resistance. Within six months this otherwise cooperative patient was viewed as totally noncompliant and irascible.

Kaplan De-Nour concludes from her own work that staff judges patients as if they were a homogenous group whose behavior should be stable over time. The critical issue is staff criteria for judging a patient to be noncompliant. Borkman (1976) notes that staff makes relatively quick judgments of patients' intelligence, relating it to compliance (i.e., higher intelligence–higher compliance rate). Kaplan De-Nour writes that the noncompliant patient is viewed as troublesome, unlikeable, of lower intelligence, and medically more unstable. Gerber (1980) examined staff versus patient perception of loss or changes after going on chronic dialysis. Staff overemphasized the importance to patients of changes such as decreased sexual behavior and family concerns while underemphasizing losses due to dietary restriction, travel limitations, and inability to complete household chores. In short, patients' sense of life priorities was significantly different than that of the staff treating them. Patients were intensely preoccupied with a personal, day-to-day sense of productivity unrelated to their relationships to others, whereas the rating of the nurses, in turn, reflected their own personal life circumstances. From this series of studies, it can be summarized that the noncompliant patient is so designated because of value differences between staff members and the patients they judge. Patients look to medical staff for cure, but in dialysis this is not possible. Calland (1972), a physician and himself a dialysis patient, believes that this is translated into a conversation (such as the one below) that he has heard many times:

DOCTOR: (on daily rounds) How are you doing?
PATIENT: I'm feeling rotten.
DOCTOR: You're doing just fine.

The patient retreats after such dialogue, realizing that his complaints are probably not treatable but are the expected side effects of the dialysis. The dialogue reflects the staff's denial of the subjective experience of the patient (i.e., the patient's perception of his quality of life). The physician knows that little can be offered for many of his patients' chronic complaints. Kaplan De-Nour and Czaczkes (1974) found that nephrologists overestimate patient compliance as a way of coping with their own high stress level due to the difficulty of treating such patients. With the dialysis patient, many dietary restrictions are ignored within a certain margin of noncompliance within which the patient knows he is safe. Although given stern warning by well-meaning staff to forego vegetables with high potassium levels, H.B., a patient on dialysis for six years, continued to eat lettuce daily. When confronted with high blood chemistries, he said that he knew he could eat a certain amount of lettuce with no resulting physical discomfort. Seime (1980) has studied the relationship between noncompliance and resulting symptomatology in dialysis patients. Over a three-month period, he analyzed objective indicators of noncompliance in three patients and their self-report of symptoms. Results showed that there was no clear relationship between symptoms (e.g., feeling poorly) and compliance indicators (e.g., fluid overload). Noncompliance did not make patients feel bad in the short run. Feeling poorly at some later time was not attributed to noncompliance but rather was seen as the result of the overall disease process. Blodgett's (1981) work also supports the idea that patients invariably abuse their diet and operate within individual parameters of safe noncompliance. Such behavior reflects the notion of Anger and Anger (1976) that all dialysis patients have an understandable ambivalence toward living on dialysis and that noncompliance is one mode of attempting to continue living a normal life.

Research indicates (Gerber, 1984) that staff ratings of patients' adjustment to dialysis are a function of the quality of the relationship between staff and the patient rated, rather than objective assessments. Kaplan De-Nour and Czaczkes (1974) observe that the intensive, chronic nature of the dialysis regimen promotes the formation of close staff–patient relationships which heightens the emotional investment of staff and patient in one another. Furthermore, staff ratings of patient noncompliance tend to be global and do not take into account the fact that patients can be noncompliant with one aspect of the regimen yet compliant with another. The case of a 40-year-old dialysis patient illustrates the latter: S.E. had been on dialysis for 27 months when the consulting psychologist was asked to see him because he was noncompliant. After a thorough psychological assessment, his case was reviewed in a multidisciplinary meeting. It became apparent that, while the patient followed his dietary regimen closely, he was less compulsive about taking his phosphate-binding medication as prescribed, resulting in abnormal calcium blood levels. The psychologist, who was unfamiliar with dialysis, soon learned that medication was in the form of a very large pill taken up to twelve times per day. The staff was reluctant to view the patient's behavior as being basically noncompliant. Although the medication's value is indisputable, the patient stated that the pill was large and dissolved slowly, leaving an unpleasant taste throughout the day. Moreover, the eventual negative effects of taking fewer tablets were, even the physician would admit, off somewhere in the future. For S.E., as with many patients, dialysis, unrealistically, alters his sense of the importance of the distant future. He chose—with full awareness—to lessen present aversive consequences, though his otherwise rational behavior might appear noncompliant. This case also serves to illustrate the problems with the term often used to explain noncompliance in dialysis patients—denial. The term denial has a strong negative quality to it, rooted in its original psychoanalytical context as one of the basic defenses against the conscious recognition of unpleasant thoughts, memories, and feelings. When denial is used to understand an individual's behavior, it has a judgmental tone which implies that if the individual does not behave the way he is expected to, he cannot tolerate some aspect of reality (i.e., so he denies that aspect). Thus, in the above example if the choice of S.E. not to take the medication is viewed as the product of an unconcious process (i.e., denial), it implies that there is something wrong with the patient—he is denying reality. Actually, the patient's behavior is the result of a conscious choice of one behavior over another. Staff interject the question, "If he chooses not to take the medicine, then isn't he denying the seriousness of his illness?" Denial here is used to minimize the patient's different perspective on his situation, a perspective differing from the staff. The logic of concluding that if someone doesn't do what others think best then he is showing psychopathology, is a classic bind that does not serve the patient's real interest. Early reports on noncompliance in dialysis patients used denial as a central explanatory mechanism (Goldstein, 1972). More recent articles (Kaplan De-Nour, 1982) have minimized the importance of patient denial in determining noncompliant behavior while emphasizing the unresponsiveness of the staff to real patient concerns.

Compliance: The Ultimate Dilemma of the Dialysis Patient

The staff's assumption that a patient should be totally aware of his condition and all its medical and psychological implications is clearly unrealistic. Such a notion represents the projection of medical staff who, indeed, should be aware of the implications of the diseases the staff treats. The patient's constant awareness, however, serves little useful purpose, particularly in a situation in which the most perfectly compliant patient will still not be able to reverse his condition. This facet, unique to the chronically ill patient, is a major psychological contributor to that behavior called noncompliance. Here, the issues of control and influence are paramount. The patient is asked to exercise extreme self-discipline but with no possibility of his medical condition improving. Staff request the patient to be future-oriented when his life expectancy is undoubtedly foreshortened. Patients are asked to lead normal lives when, in fact, their life circumstances on dialysis are truly extraordinary. Research evidence supports the idea that medical staff have unrealistically high expectations of dialysis patients, (Kaplan De-Nour & Czaczkes, 1974). One physician interviewed by these authors in their 1974 study believed that all dialysis patients should be relaxed on dialysis, and others believed that the patients should feel no weakness. The authors comment, "Is it realistic to expect patients with a hematocrit around 20 percent not to feel a permanent weakness or is that another sign of the physician's inability to accept life on dialysis as not so easy and pleasant?" (p. 221). In addition, staff members who regularly work with dialysis patients will agree that, not infrequently, patients considered to be compliant die much sooner and unexpectedly than do the uncooperative patients. An example is S.J.

> S.J. was a 60-year-old patient who had been on the machine for eleven years. He was considered to be the most noncompliant patient in our large center's 12-year history. S.J. was obese, a long-term diabetic, and legally blind. He lived off of a small monthly social security check. He was usually late for treatments, sometimes skipping treatments altogether. He regularly showed dangerously high potassium, occasionally over 8 meq/L (7 meq/L is considered lethal). His fluid gain between

dialysis sessions was usually in excess of three kilos, occasionally as high as 10 kilos. He also demanded to be taken off dialysis after three hours instead of four. He constantly took unprescribed medication while taking prescribed medication in amounts either too small or too large. His demeanor was usually unpleasant and angry. In weekly meetings with the unit psychologist, nurses shared with each other their great frustration about this patient's behavior. While S.J. lived a completely noncompliant lifestyle in his 10 years of dialyzing, scores of patients, labeled compliant, expired. The nurses struggled with what they considered to be the injustice of this situation. S.J. answered that he would do what he wanted and didn't care how long he lived.

This dubious correlation between chronic noncompliance and longer survival on dialysis is illustrated in hundreds of other cases. It reflects the complex physical factors that are beyond the scope of medicine to predict or control satisfactorily. Thus, patients realize that neither compliance nor noncompliance to the prescribed regimen offers any certain outcome. Patients remark that they see no reason to be unfailingly compliant.

We have outlined the specifics of the dialysis regimen and the issue of compliance in this population. However, the experience of dialysis illuminates psychological phenomena pertinent to other chronic illnesses. Although the specific physical consequences of chronic renal failure are unique to that condition, the psychological implications of the disease's many restrictions are similar to those of other chronic illnesses (Burish & Bradley, 1983). A variety of chronic illnesses (e.g., diabetes, arthritis, hypertension) demand serious life changes similar to those of the dialysis patient. Compliance with diet, medication and level of activity recommendations are endemic to the chronically ill. The familial, interpersonal, vocational, and phenomenological impact described in regard to the dialysis patient would be true—to some degree, lesser or greater—for most chronic illnesses. In addition, medical progress ensures that soon other machinery will be regularly used to keep alive patients who now die from a variety of end-stage organ failure. We might expect that the complications of being kept alive by a dialysis machine will be limited in these future patient groups. What are some solutions to this prevalent problem of noncompliance?

Traditional Behavioral Approaches to Noncompliance

Psychologists have often proposed a behavioral (operant) treatment of noncompliance. This model has been suggested for use with the dialysis population (Goldstein & Fenster, 1973). Prompting and contracting are examples of operant approaches. More recently proposed broad spectrum behavioral techniques include biofeedback and hypnosis and are used for a variety of compliance problems in the chronically ill (i.e., lessening stressful responses will help a patient cope better). In our view, such clinical strategies are often short-sighted and in the actual clinical environment will fail over the long run. Unlike more comprehensive behavioral models (cf. Chapter 4 of this book), these traditional psychological approaches fail to consider the true experimental parameters of being a dialysis patient. Yalom (1980) has written of the relevance of certain philosophical concerns to the practice of traditional psychotherapy. Such concerns are no less relevant to the psychologist working with the noncompliant chronically ill patient. Although philosophical ideas do not easily translate into clinical practice, such notions provide needed impetus to understanding the true concerns of the patient. Meichenbaum (Meichenbaum & Gilmore, 1982) a respected behavioral theorist, has widened the notion of the acceptable focus of the therapeutic relationship. Specifically, he writes that understanding the phenomenological experience of the patient is critical to successful treatment. The patient's "current concerns" (i.e., implicit beliefs, values) must be addressed if we are to understand the noncompliant behavior of the chronically ill patient. With this understanding, we can design appropriate treatment strategies. Without this understanding, typical behavioral treatment for noncompliance, in our experience, is fruitless. The following case illustrates this phenomenon.

C.T., a 52-year-old veteran, was on dialysis for three months when a consultant was asked to evaluate his noncompliance to diet and fluid intake restrictions. The patient was an unstable diabetic with severe retinopathy and a left leg amputation. During the interview he remarked that he was tired of the restrictions imposed by both diabetes and chronic renal failure. He appeared anxious and depressed. The psychologist offered some emotional support and designed a behavioral intervention to increase compliant behaviors. The plan consisted of relaxation training coupled with autogenic exercises to reduce anxiety. Contingency contracting was also devised whereby strict dietary adherence was to be rewarded by weekend trips in which the patient had expressed interest. Staff was asked to ignore the patient's "negative" behavior in favor of responding to any compliant or positive behaviors he showed. This treatment protocol produced some immediate increase in compliance to diet but no change in regard to fluid intake. Depression and anxiety remained high. Within three months, C.T. was at the same point as prior to the psychologist's evaluation.

Noncompliance as an Attempted Solution to the Existential Crisis

The operant treatment model, in essence, a technological one, failed because it did not consider that the patient's behavior was, in a very real sense, an attempt to solve the existential issues for which there are no pat answers. Patients such as C.T. need not be persuaded that compliance is important or that they are responsible for their behavior. On closer examination, certain facts stood out in C.T.'s case. He was an Italian-American with a strong sense of responsibility for and leadership within his family. His physical limitations prevented him from exercising the role he had assumed for many years. Food was also critical to him, and he had long prided himself on his cooking Italian delicacies. He was no longer capable of cooking intricate dishes. He spent much of his out-of-bed time sitting on his back porch. He was unable to garden—his favorite avocation—because of his blindness and weakness. He developed chronic diarrhea as a complication of diabetes. He saw this as a humiliating and greatly limiting problem. His physical condition was irreversibly downhill, yet perhaps years away from final resolution. He viewed, though poorly articulated, the behavioral techniques as superficial and "not for someone in my situation." He expressed a profound feeling of alienation from others to whom he had previously been close. His sense of worth and his definition of himself had changed, for which he could see no remedy. His sense of purpose and responsibility for his circumstances had been radically altered by his chronic disease. Compliance was futile, even trivial, to the patient. Staff judgments of the patient alternated between sympathy and anger. C.T. insisted on bringing into the dialysis unit his own lunch which usually consisted of some foods he knew were forbidden. Staff would angrily confront him with this fact but to no avail. Here the ideas of Abrams (1974) are relevant. In the earliest days of dialysis treatment, he suggested that staff must be open to a patient telling us—directly or through his behavior—that life has become intolerable. To assume that all patients can see the value in life that we strive to preserve is an expression of the staff's own wish for omnipotence and immortality. If noncompliance is simply a function of lack of information or poor structuring of time and activity (i.e., not planning grocery shopping, thereby making it "necessary" to eat in a restaurant where food is more likely to be not allowed on the diet), such a technological strategy may suffice. In our clinical work with patients such as C.T., we have seen the technician's approach fail—almost without exception.

As an alternative, the following approach was taken with C.T.: A psychologist spent frequent but brief sessions with him exploring his premorbid history and present situation. His current concerns and the desperation of his situation were openly discussed. His family was called in, and C.T. shared with them many of the concerns he had been unable to express previously. His family, with the help of the psychologist, began to appreciate the patient's sense of loss and futility. His behavior became understandable, and they were less inclined to criticize or police him as before. A priest was summoned and visited the patient frequently. Within the context of this broader approach, concrete suggestions were made regarding time usage. However, goals to enhance compliance were set aside in favor of supportive counseling and modifying staff expectations. As family communication improved and staff pressure subsided, patient compliance also improved, if somewhat slightly. Affect showed noticeable positive change, although a withdrawn demeanor was present much of the time.

Rather than being "an immovable factor" (Zifferblatt, 1975), the existential concerns of the patient often are the fundamental dynamism without which behavior change techniques are futile.

In her provocative essay on how aloneness and the need for

solitude complicates the compliance issue, Purtillo (1980) also rails against the philosophy of adherence technology which holds that compliance problems in the last analysis can always be reduced to behavioral problems. In recounting an episode of noncompliance on the part of one of her patients, Purtillo puts it this way: "It was only some years later that I remembered the incident and realized that he was crying for a moment of solitude and we, the well-intentioned health professionals, were offering the sponge of *loneliness* in its place" (p. 93).

In our view, a fundamental paradox (and irony of our modern technological age) resides in the attempt to apply a strict behavioral methodology to secure a patient's participation or persuade the patient of the importance of adherence to the requisite regimen when his pattern of noncompliance represents an attempted solution to a series of existential crises.

THE CANCER CLINIC: WHERE COMPLIANCE IS TAKEN SERIOUSLY

Cancer patients who come for chemotherapy have the highest rate of compliance with the treatment regimen and all that it demands of any group of patients under treatment for serious medical problems at the Long Beach VA Medical Center. As noncompliance thrives in virtually all of the other general medical and specialty clinics throughout the hospital, the question arises: Why is the problem almost nonexistent in this group of patients?[1]

This phenomenon is all the more curious and intriguing when one reflects upon the miseries often associated with chemotherapy and the demands placed on these patients for proper compliance with the regimen. Discomfort, nausea, and vomiting occur during or after the actual infusion or injection of the chemotherapy in some 50 percent of the cases. Patients must often comply with taking medicine as prescribed. Patients on the small cell lung cancer protocol not only have to come to the hospital for four days every three weeks but also must return to clinic every week for laboratory studies, complete a 24-hour urine collection every three weeks, and every three months maintain a detailed food diary for three days at a time. Chemotherapy patients taking procarbazine must, in addition, adhere to dietary and alcohol restrictions.

While the reasons for such a high rate of compliance are surely multifaceted and complex, the psychological motivation for such extraordinary compliance would seem to involve three experiential aspects.

The Pressure of Time

A striking difference between the cancer patient on chemotherapy and the end-stage renal disease patient on dialysis rests not only with the absolute amount of time that lies ahead, but, more importantly, with their perception of the time remaining in their lives. The epithet "the too-long life" suggests the dialysis patient perceives time as moving slowly—a perception that is affectively unpleasant and that precludes the phenomenological expectation of future changes. By contrast, the cancer patient, with extensive disease and cognizant of his prognosis, must feel the pressure of time intensely and perceive time as moving swiftly. Decisions to embark upon a demanding course of treatment and to comply faithfully with its requirements are made against a backdrop of the moving hands of the clock and for this reason are made, perhaps, more easily.

Exorcism and the Struggle Against the Tumor: Good Versus Evil

A second motivation for the chemotherapy patient's remarkably conscientious adherence to the treatment regimen may lie in the nature of the disease. One commonality of the insidious collection of diseases known as cancer, not true of other serious, chronic, incurable, often fatal illnesses such as endstage renal disease, diabetes, or heart disease is that cancer always involves something foreign growing unpredictably in one's body—sometimes chaotically, sometimes insidiously. In the provocative phrase of Avery Weisman (1979), it resembles the crab that creeps along quietly with claws reaching out in all directions and is evocative of primitive fears and superstitions. Kidney failure, diabetes, and coronary heart disease, on the other hand, involve nothing foreign to the body, only the malfunction or wearing out of the body's own organs.

Cancer, unlike other diseases, is evocative of an evil malediction and is symbolic of social ills. In some circles it remains a taboo topic and is still regarded as a peculiar stigma—like the leprosy of ancient times or the Plague of medieval times. The folly and tragedy of this attitude is nowhere more dramatically apparent than in modern day Greece where a pervasive cultural denial has conditioned the attitudes of its people. Uterine cancer must be euphemistically characterized as "adhesions", lung cancer as "a shadow on the lung," gastric carcinomas are "ulcers—bad ulcers," and treatment (radiotherapy) becomes diathermy. Physicians in Greece have actually met their death at the hands of irate families for having told their relatives they had cancer.

Thus, the patient's fight against cancer may unconsciously invoke a struggle against evil, summoning an individual rallying cry, a mobilization of individual resources not seen in diabetes or renal disease, in the hope of exorcism.

The Chance for Cure: Magic and the Psychology of Beating the Odds

Patients buffer themselves against the reality of death by a variety of defense mechanisms and coping strategies. Society obliges with ready-made patterns of rationalization in the form of religious belief systems which are invariably characterized by magic and regression. Resorting to magic can occur on a more personalized level as well. Through an idealization of one's doctors and their instructions which are carefully obeyed, the patient can cherish a belief in the magic power of his treatment. The belief that one is an exception is a common human trait.

In Gullo's (1973) description of the death denier—the dying child who admits both to his illness and its gravity but insists that he will be "one of the lucky statistics" who can beat the odds—we glimpse part of the psychological motivation of the adult who is offered chemotherapy. When the patient with small cell cancer of the lung and limited disease is told that the odds are 80 percent that he will respond to therapy, with a reduction in the size of the tumor, that chemotherapy can prolong his life up to two years and that there is a 20 percent chance of extending his life three years or longer—with such prognostications, he takes refuge in the magical thinking of the unconscious, believing that he will be the one to beat the odds. The patient translates the oncologist's rational statement of probabilities into the wishful illusion of the bettor: "I will be the one to beat the odds . . . ."

A Special Case of Noncompliance

Compliance with the treatment regimen necessitates an implicit doctor-patient "contract." Whether this contract fits a paternalistic model of a fiduciary contract or a negotiated mutual contract is immaterial. The doctor-patient relationship is based fundamentally on a *contract* that may or may not assume an underlying equality between patient and physician. The patient, in any event, has contracted for medical services with some implicit verbal agreement (i.e., informed consent)—at least at the outset—to the regimen of prescribed medical care.

What about the cancer patient who disengages entirely from the medical care contract? Oncologists will, infrequently, encounter patients who have completed a partial series of chemotherapy and in the midst of their course of treatment decide they wish to forego further treatment and terminate their medical care. A conservative estimate places their number at between two and four percent of the total population of cancer patients served at the Long Beach VA Medical Center[2] and less than two percent of private patients.[3] About half of these elect to pursue a nonconventional treatment (e.g., laetril or immunotherapy), and the remaining few are lost to follow up with their reasons and subsequent history unknown and unknowable.

A thoughtful, though perhaps not reasoned, decision to terminate treatment, which is not reached precipitously, in an otherwise compliant cancer patient with advanced, noncurable disease may not be viewed universally as noncompliance. Nonetheless, the patient who decides to terminate treatment and any further contact is, in effect if not in fact, totally rejecting the best advice and the regimen worked out for him by the physicians in whom he has entrusted his care. In this definitional sense, stopping treatment is the ultimate act of noncompliance.

Whether this set of events is properly termed noncompliant behavior is perhaps debatable. To put it another way, for someone with advanced, noncurable disease, unswerving compliance to an arduous regimen of chemotherapy, the state of the art such as it is, may not be the healthiest choice or in the patient's best interest. In short, while this could be considered a special form of noncompliance, it may be a legitimate one. Parenthetically, a test of this issue might be determined by the question: Will the treatment preserve and/or enhance life, as in the case of the patient under treatment for high blood pressure or diabetes, or only prolong their life—read, misery, in the case of the cancer patient who will certainly die of the disease within the not too distant future?

When Death Is Imminent

Our discussion of compliance in the cancer patient would not be complete without mention of that rare instance of less-than-perfect compliance that is observed in the terminal patient. Wright and Nehemkis (1983) describe a case in which the apparent noncompliance involved the patient's obsessive preoccupation with relatively minor, secondary physical manifestations of the cancer rather than with the disease itself, resulting in a series of delaying tactics to forestall the resumption of regularly scheduled cycles of chemotherapy. In sum, for this patient, to accept treatment was tantamount to accepting cancer, while refusing treatment was a rejection of the existence of cancer.

What appears to be a form of noncompliance—temporarily refusing chemotherapy—is not, upon closer examination, what is generally meant by the term. Unless the meaning of the term noncompliance is stretched so as to encompass manifestations of death anxiety and fear of death in dying patients, the preceding illustrative case is not properly labeled as noncompliance. Those relatively infrequent instances of less-than-perfect compliance observed among terminal cancer patients are best understood as providing a focal point by which they can divert attention from their underlying fears and protect themselves against the psychological threatening losses and changes that signal impending death. In such a case, the question of noncompliance is really moot, for two reasons: (1) death is imminent, and (2) because of the nearness of death, there is virtually no likelihood that the patient's behavior one way or the other will affect the outcome.

REFERENCE NOTES

1. Ulmer, R. A. *Noncompliance problems of cancer patients and their resolution.* Unpublished manuscript, Martin Luther King, Jr. General Hospital, 1980. The statistics cited by Ulmer, for example, placing the percentage of noncompliant cancer patients at 25 percent are general, i.e., span all seven phases of cancer management (1. prevention, 2. detection, 3. diagnosis, 4. pretreatment, 5. treatment, 6. rehabilitation, 7. continuing care) and cannot be clearly interpreted for that subset of patients already under treatment or continuing care. Thus, it is not clear from these pooled data whether the percentages are indeed significantly inconsistent from our own.

2. Kasimis, Basil, M.D. and Claudia Kaneshiro, Pharm. D., Hematology-Oncology Section, Long Beach VA Medical Center. Personal Communication, December, 1982.

3. Fass, Leroy, M.D., Oncologist in private practice, Memorial Hospital Medical Center, Long Beach, California. Personal Communication, February, 1983.

REFERENCES

Abram, H. The psychiatrist, the treatment of chronic renal failure, and the prolongation of life: I. *American Journal of Psychiatry, 124*, 1351–1358, 1968.

Abram, H. The psychiatrist, the treatment of chronic renal failure, and the prolongation of life: II. *American Journal of Psychiatry, 126*, 157–167, 1969.

Abram, H. The "uncooperative" hemodialysis patient. In N. B. Levy (Ed), *Living or dying.* New York: Wiley, 1974.

Abram, H. Psychiatry and medical progress: Therapeutic considerations. *International Journal of Psychiatry in Medicine, 6*, 203–211, 1975.

Alexander, L. The double-bind theory and hemodialysis. *Archives of General Psychiatry, 33*, 1353–1356, 1976.

Anger, D., & Anger, D. W. Dialysis ambivalence: A matter of life and death. *American Journal of Nursing, 76*, 276–277, 1976.

Armstrong, S. H. Psychological maladjustment in renal dialysis patients. *Psychosomatic Medicine, 19*, 169–171, 1978.

Armstrong, S. H. The common structure of treatment staff attitudes toward adolescent dialysis patients. *Psychotherapy and Psychosomatics, 26*, 322–329, 1975.

Benjamin, D. CAPD didn't work for me. *NAPHT News*, 6–7, February 1983.
Blodgett, C. A selected review of the literature of adjustment to hemodialysis. *International Journal of Psychiatry and Medicine*, *11*, 97–124, 1981–1982.
Borkman, T. Hemodialysis compliance: The relationship of staff estimates of patients' intelligence and understanding to compliance. *Social Science and Medicine*, *10*, 385–392, 1976.
Burton, H., Canzons, L., Wall, L. Holden, R., Conley, J., & Lindsay, R. Life without the machine: A look at the psychological determinants for successful adaptation of patients on CAPD. In N. Levy (Ed.), *Psycho-Nephrology* 2. New York: Plenum, 1983.
Calland, C. Iatrogenic problems in end stage renal failure. *New England Journal of Medicine*, *287*, 334–336, 1972.
Gerber, K. Staff vs. patient perceptions of life change in hemodialysis patients. Paper presented at the Eleventh Annual Meeting of the Western Dialysis and Transplant Society, San Francisco, 1980.
Gerber, K., Falke, R., Ralidis, P. Social support and compliance to medical regimen in hemodialysis patients. Paper presented at the 64th Annual Meeting of the Western Psychological Association, Los Angeles, 1984.
Goldstein, A. Denial and external locus of control as mechanisms of adjustment in chronic medical illness. *Essence*, *1*, 5–22, 1976.
Goldstein, A. The subjective experience of denial in an objective investigation of chronically ill patients. *Psychosomatics*, *13*, 20–22, 1972.
Goldstein, A., & Fenster, C. A. The role of the mental health practitioner in long term medical treatment. *Psychosomatics*, *14*, 153–155, 1973.
Gullo, S. V. Games children play when they're dying. *Medical Dimensions*, *2*, 23–28, 1973.
Hartman, P. E., & Becker, M. H. Noncompliance with prescribed regimen among chronic hemodialysis patients: A method of prediction and educational diagnosis. *Dialysis and Transplantation*, *7*, 978–989, 1978.
Kaplan De-Nour, A. Staff-patient interaction. In N. Levy (Ed.), *Psycho-Nephrology* 2. New York: Plenum, 1982.
Kaplan De-Nour, A., & Czaczkes, J. W. Personality factors in chronic hemodialysis patients causing noncompliance with medical regimen. *Psychosomatic Medicine*, *34*, 333–344, 1972.
Kaplan De-Nour, A., & Czaczkes, J. W. Bias in assessment of patients on chronic dialysis. *Journal of Psychosomatic Research*, *18*, 217–221, 1974.
Kaplan De-Nour, A., & Czaczkes, J. W. Personality and adjustment to chronic hemodialysis. In N. B. Levy (Ed.), *Living or dying: Adaptation to hemodialysis*. Springfield, IL: Charles C Thomas, 1974.
Kaplan De-Nour, A., & Czaczkes, J. W. The influence of patient's personality on adjustment to chronic dialysis. *Journal of Nervous and Mental Disorders*, *162*, 323–333, 1976.
Meichenbaum, D., & Gilmore, J. B. Resistance from a cognitive-behavioral perspective. In P. Wachtel (Ed.), *Resistance: Psychodynamic and behavioral approaches*. New York, Plenum Press, 1982.
Purtillo, R. B. Loneliness, the need for solitude, and compliance. In D. J. Withersty, J. M. Stevenson, & R. H. Waldman (Eds.), *Communication and compliance in a hospital setting*. New York: Charles C Thomas, 1980.

Schulz, K., & Aderman, D. How the medical staff copes with dying patients: A critical review. *Omega, 7*, 11–21, 1976.

Seime, R. J. The relationship of compliance, self-reported feelings and symptoms, and staff attention in dialysis: A pilot study. In D. J. Withersty, J. M. Stevenson, & R. H. Waldman (Eds.), *Communication and compliance in a hospital setting.* New York: Charles C Thomas, 1980.

Streltzer, J., Markhoff, R., & Yano, B. Maintenance hemodialysis in patients with pre-existing psychiatric disorders. *Journal of Nervous and Mental Disorders, 164*, 414–418, 1977.

Viederman, M. On the vicissitudes of the need for control in patients confronted with hemodialysis. *Comprehensive Psychiatry, 19*, 455–467, 1978.

Weatzel, N., Vollrath, D., Ritz, E., & Ferner, H. Analysis of patient-nurse interaction in hemodialysis units. *Journal of Psychosomatic Research, 21*, 359–366, 1977.

Weisman, A. *Coping with cancer.* New York: McGraw-Hill, 1979.

Wright, M. & Nehemkis, A. Functional use of secondary cancer symptomatology. *International Journal of Psychiatry in Medicine, 13*(4), 267–275, 1983–1984.

Wright, R., Sand, P., & Livingston, G. Psychological stress during hemodialysis for chronic renal failure. *Annals of Internal Medicine, 64*, 611–621, 1966.

Yalom, I. D. *Existential psychotherapy.* New York: Basic Books, 1980.

Yanadiga, E. H., & Streltzer, J. Limitations of psychological tests in a dialysis population. *Psychosomatic Medicine, 41*, 557–567, 1979.

Zaner, R. Dialysis and ethics: Be strong and trust (please!) In N. Levy (Ed.), *PsychoNephrology I.* New York: Plenum, 1981.

Zifferblatt, S. M. Increasing patient compliance through the applied analysis of behavior. *Preventive Medicine, 4*, 173–182, 1975.

6

Family Relationships
and Compliance

Amy Herstein Gervasio

Family relationships are often cited but seldom studied as important components of the chronically ill patient's compliance with medical regimen. Litman (1974) argued a decade ago that the family is the "basic unit" of health care; yet the functioning of that unit in obtaining and carrying out treatment of chronic illness remains inadequately addressed. Many researchers note that although a host of studies relate compliance to family demographics and role relationships, a coherent sociological or psychological theory of family dynamics in the context of chronic illness has yet to be advanced (Becker & Green, 1975; DiMatteo & DiNichola, 1982; Litman & Venters, 1979). In the absence of such a theory, the different perspectives, measures, and results of these groups studies cannot be synthesized into a complete account of how families support and hinder compliance with treatment programs.

Traditionally viewed as the primary focus of treatment, the individual patient has until recently been taken as the proper focus of compliance studies as well. Researchers seeking to expand that focus must turn to the field of family therapy, which like many other areas in sociology and psychology, lacks a clearly superior school of theory and treatment (Gurman & Kniskern, 1981). The field itself cannot offer an approach for assessing family functioning that is at once widely recognized, highly reliable, and comprehensive. Occupational biases also inhibit an integration of approaches. Family therapists who work with the chronically ill often concentrate on understanding the functions that illness and treatment serve in the ongoing dynamics of specific families (cf. Cohen & Wellisch, 1978; Herz, 1980; Slivkin, 1977). Therefore, they are more inclined to report individual case studies than to compile and analyze group data. Sociologists and social psychologists who use experimental methods tend to study factors such as the health attitudes of the family that distinguish noncompliant from compliant groups. The difficult task of linking group tendencies to the individual family's process of coping with illness is generally evaded by researchers of either discipline.

Despite limited theoretical and empirical attention, family relationships and compliance have gained increasing recognition as an important practical axis for viewing the delivery of health care. This chapter presents an overview of the kinds of research that have examined the impact of family relationships on compliance, a brief overview of psychoanalytic, behavioral, and systems approaches to the family, and case studies illustrating how systems views of family functioning may be applied to various problems in compliance.

RESEARCH

The earliest and most prevalent type of research regarding the family's impact on health care relates demographic variables (such as socioeconomic status, education, occupation, leisure time, age, sex, and number of family members) to utilization of medical services, medication, preventive health programs, and compliance. Most of these studies use hospital records and large-scale surveys. By these methods, Muller (1965) and Tucker (1970), for example, found support for the claim that people of lower socioeconomic status are less likely to have access to and use medical services. Occasionally, demographic data permits researchers to challenge common sense assumptions. One such assumption might be that divorced families are weaker units of care than intact families. Wingert, Larson, and Friedman (1968), however, found that intact and broken families were equally likely to use emergency medical services when their children were ill. Their results suggest that nontraditional family structures may possess hidden (i.e., unassumed) strengths.

The main service performed by demographic research is the isolation of those broad variables that merit closer inquiry by other methods. In a study of the relationship of family demographic variables to individual medicine use, Osterweis, Bush, and Zuckerman (1979) isolated several family characteristics that compliance research might pursue. They found that overall family morbidity was a better predictor of medicine use than the health of individual members; that when there were more children in the family, the family was likely to use more nonprescription drugs; and that the percentage of females in the family was inversely related to the use of prescribed medicine and directly related to the use of over-the-counter drugs. Such correlations alert researchers to important roles family members and characteristics might play in the individual patient's compliance, but cannot specify *how* those roles are played.

Role Relationships

Research on family relationships appears to be the most relevant to family impact on compliance. As Litman and Venters (1979) observe, studies in this area are few and often methodologically flawed. Many of the measures they use are of questionable validity, typically depending upon self-report questionnaires. Families are seldom studied *in vivo*. Instead, relationships and roles are inferred from responses to a few questionnaire items. Some studies gather information about the roles of all family members from one member exclusively. Although flawed and limited in scope, the literature tends to support the claim that roles in the family have a bearing on the compliance of patients.

Some researchers have focused on particular members' influence on the family's use of health services. Baric (1970) studied the husband's influence on the use of preventive health services by the wife. He addressed husbands by letters that urged them to encourage their wives to have pap smears and found that the letters did not affect the likelihood that the wives would make appointments. However, wives in marriages with "merged/coopera-tive roles" (according to a self-report measure of decision making) were more likely to use health services. In another study of couples' attitudes toward preventive health, Becker, Kaback, Rosenstock, and Ruth (1975) found that the convergence and similarity of spouses' beliefs about their susceptibility to, and the severity of, Tay-Sachs disease predicted the likelihood of their using screening facilities. In a study by Aho (1977), cardiac patients' wives who strongly endorsed belief statements indicating that spouses could play a role in prevention and treatment of heart disease were in fact more likely to propose behavior changes to their own husbands than wives who responded less confidently.

After completing a three generational analysis of family members' health habits, Litman (1974, p. 505) concluded that the wife-mother "remains the central agent of cure and care within the family complex". The wife-mother visits doctors more often and takes more medication than other family members. Litman (1974) postulates that the wife-mother needs to take more medication because she is reluctant to assume a sick role; her absence from her usual duties is less tolerated by the family than the father's absence. He found that the traditional family became more disorganized during the mother's sickness than during the father's because it lost its housekeeper and prime source of nurturance (Litman, 1971). Small families experienced more role reversal and shift than large ones, because in large families the older children—especially the daughters—assumed the mother's role. Litman (1971) argues that the small, close family may also be severely strained by one member's chronic illness, whereas a large, less close family may have learned to deal with stresses, strains, and absences. In either family type, the mother assumes an extra burden when she takes care of ill grand-parents, a burden likely to strain her psychological and physical resources. Finally, Litman (1971) found little evidence to show that the relation of family health habits to the wife-mother role was different for "egalitarian" versus "maternally dominated" families. It is possible that research conducted in the 1980s would show such a difference; however, true egalitarianism is probably still rare. In any case, Litman's work runs counter to the proverbial wisdom that "illness brings the family closer together"; he notes that illness is equally likely to pull the family further apart.

The mother's role seems important in the family's adjustment to terminal as well as acute illness. Cohen, Dizenhuz, and Winget (1977) found that families behaved differently toward terminally ill women than terminally ill men. Among other findings, they report that females were not told about terminality as often as men. They also found significant correlations between the effective adjustment of families after the death of a member and the surviving members' abilities to communicate with one another and to share information and decision making. Families whose terminal patient was the mother were rated significantly lower in ability to communicate than families in which the father had died. In addition, families in which the mother had died reported more difficulty in managing household tasks. Presumably, the remaining members require not only homemaking skills but also a family communicator to relegate such tasks.

Findings on role relationships suggest that the wife-mother role may be the crucial one for compliance in cases of chronic illness; however, her role has yet to be studied in that context.

Family Support

Although it seems obvious that the support of the family would be a major factor in compliance and recovery, few studies have examined family support in a systematic manner (DiMatteo & Hays, 1981). Oakes (1970) found a direct relationship between patients' use of a handsplint for arthritis and their perceptions of whether the family members strongly expected the patients to wear it. Diamond, Weiss, and Grynbaum (1968) note that the family's positive attitude toward rehabilitation is the most important factor in determining the patient's participation in spinal cord rehabilitation and compliance with physical therapy.

Green, Levine, and Wolle (1979) found that 70 percent of outpatients with primary hypertension reported that their families lacked both understanding of the disease and support for maintaining compliance with medical regimen. These researchers created a patient-education program, including home visits by staff, to encourage family support. The program enhanced patient compliance with medication but demonstrated only a moderate effect on weight loss. In a similar vein, Heinzelmann and Bagley (1970) found that a wife's attitudes toward preventive health programs for heart disease predicted her husband's level of compliance with a special preventive health activity program.

DiMatteo and Hays (1981) note that family support may have negative consequences for some patients. Feeling overwhelmed by, or burdensome to, their families may cause patients to minimize symptoms or reject care.

Family Dynamics

Several studies have attempted to relate family dynamics to compliance. Steidl, Finkelstein, Wexler, Feigenbaum, Kitsen, Kliger, and Quinlan (1980) videotaped 23 dialysis patients and their families during structured interviews encompassing problem-solving tasks similar to those used in studies of family interaction. The videotapes were rated by independent observers on variables such as "coalition and alignments," "expression of thoughts and feelings," and "leadership." Global assessment of family functioning did not differentiate between families with compliant and noncompliant members, but five specific family variables did. Greater adherence was found in families when the adults exhibited shared leadership, maintained a strong parental coalition, and took individual responsibility for their actions. These family members had open responses to the opinions of others and demonstrated effective problem-solving skills. However, objective measures of overall physical health were not related to adherence. These findings reaffirm the fact that a support network may have a direct influence on compliance, but that compliance by itself is not the only factor in physical health.

In another study of dialysis patients, MacElveen (1972) asked the patient, spouse, and primary member of the health care team (a group she called the "triad") to rate levels of cooperation, trust, and perceived mutuality of common treatment goals. She found that adherence to medical regimen was related to perceptions of cooperation in the triad, to the degree of activity undertaken by the patient, and to morale as rated by other staff members. Finally, Weber (1981) found that dialysis patients in "open, healthy relationships" were more likely to be in better health than those with conflicting relationships.

When studying families with hemophiliac children, Salk, Hilgartner, and Granich (1972) found that half of the families reported having marital difficulties, often centering around the hemophiliac child. In addition, the patients and their families had different perceptions of the impact of the child's illness on family relationships; the patients were less likely to report that they had a negative impact on their families. Differences in perception may occur because children are often shielded from their parents' quarrels. If the patients had been adults, they might have been more aware of the difficulties that illness presents for family life. In another study, Whitehead (1981) found that when mothers of hemophiliacs perceived their families as functioning well, the patients were more likely to be compliant.

For couples, long-term regimens may themselves become a source of contention. O'Brien (1979) found that families including a diabetic spouse frequently reported marital conflict over that spouse's adherence to the treatment program. Most spouses did not feel that their diabetic partner was adequately compliant. In the case of diseases like diabetes, for which an ongoing regimen is inevitable, conflicts about compliance might well become part of a couple's permanent repertoire of complaints.

Kornfeld and Siegel (1979), in a report on topics discussed in couples therapy for families with terminally ill children, found that parents tended to blame difficulties they had with their children on the illness, even when the children seemed to be entering normal developmental phases. This report suggests that the patient is often used as a scapegoat for the parents' difficulties in coming to terms with the ill child's growing up. Vogel and Bell (1968) note that scapegoating also occurs in families with chronically mentally disturbed members.

Reports on dynamics in families with chronically ill members often take the form of case studies. While such data are often presented anecdotally and are of necessity retrospective, case studies can nevertheless reveal important family mechanisms that may have a bearing on compliance. For example, Cohen and Wellisch (1978) discuss the case of a cancer patient who did not take the proper dosages of pain medication. His wife had physical control over the medication and would tell him when she thought his pain was severe enough to require it—although she would always declare that he could take the medication any time he wished. Refusing to accept the severity of her husband's condition, the wife equated the amount of pain medication he needed with his level of physical degeneration. By restricting his intake of medication, she could limit on her own acknowledgment of the cancer's progression. Obviously, a large-scale questionnaire designed to measure group variables in compliance would not reveal mechanisms of this type, which are both unacknowledged by family members and directly related to compliance with treatment. Thus, the nomothetic and idiographic approaches may both convey information essential for understanding compliance.

Finally, the reviews of Becker and Green (1975) and Becker and Maiman (1980) note that studies of family variables have shown relationships between the degree of patient compliance and family members' sympathy and encouragement, their assumption of responsibility for the sick member's care, their willingness to make necessary changes in the environment, and the compatibility of usual familial roles with the patient's new sick role. How these conditions within the family can be facilitated and hindered is open to speculation. The remainder of this chapter provides a framework for such speculation and presents cases that illustrate some relevant family dynamics.

THEORIES OF FAMILY FUNCTIONING

The majority of approaches to family therapy follow one of three orientations: psychoanalytic, behavioral, or systems. The therapeutic approaches from these orientations can be augmented by recent theoretical work on the family life cycle (Carter & McGoldrick, 1980). Proponents from each major school have applied their theories to families with chronically ill members, but compliance has been of primary interest to behavior and systems theorists. Structural family therapy is the most prominent approach that directly addresses compliance as a family issue (Minuchin & Fishman, 1981).

Psychoanalytic Views of the Family

Therapists taking psychoanalytic approaches to the family have modified concepts of traditional psychoanalysis to derive a set of basic assumptions about family dynamics. They assume that people repress unconscious conflict and childhood memories but project childhood conflict onto other family members in adulthood. The adult introjects childhood images of parental figures. Transference occurs not only between therapist and client but also between individual family members. By marrying and having children, individuals seek new resolution to old conflicts. In families with marital problems, the individuals ineffectively reconstruct their families of origin (Jones, 1980).

Psychoanalytic family therapy is often a long-term process of revealing and reworking the conflict between the individual and the family of origin (Framo, 1976). In this process, noncompliance is seen as a form of resistance, one which may signal unresolved authority conflicts between patient and doctors or between family members. The goal of psychoanalytic family therapy is to overcome such resistance and reveal the deeper conflict which symptoms like noncompliance mask. Short-term methods of enhancing compliance are of secondary importance to psychoanalytic goals and may even be seen as diverting the therapeutic process away from its primary goals. This form of therapy thus offers no specific or direct mode of treatment for noncompliance as a problem of primary importance.

Behavioral Views of the Family

Behavior therapists have developed techniques for enhancing compliance using behavioral principles of learning and reinforcement (cf. Chapter 4 of this book). Often, family members are involved in carrying out behavioral programs (cf. Dapitch–Miura & Hovell, 1979). especially when the patient is a chronically ill child. Historically, behavior therapists have concentrated on the individual patient, but some behavior theorists have recently tried to extend their theories to the family.

Family therapists in the behavioral tradition usually define the family as groups of dyads exhibiting interlocking, reciprocal behaviors (Jones, 1980; Liberman, 1972). Each individual responds habitually to other family members. Particular responses are acquired and modified through principles of learning, including operant conditioning, overt and covert modeling. Behavior is maintained or increased by reinforcers and decreased by punishers. In the operant conditioning paradigm, a reinforcer is defined as any event that both follows a response and increases the probability that the response will occur in the future. A punisher is an event which decreases the probability that the response will occur (Karoly, 1975).

Although a complete discussion of schedules of reinforcement and their impact on learning is beyond the scope of this chapter, it is important to note that social reinforcers appear to be the most powerful type of reinforcer (Patterson, 1975). However, manipulation of social reinforcers is complicated by the fact that they are *behaviors*; thus, they both effect, and are affected by, a chain of other highly probably behaviors.

Family members learn very complicated ways of responding to each other. If the behavior of an individual family member is reinforced, either purposely or accidentally, it may cause changes in the habitual behavior of other family members. "Accidental training" is a term used to describe the process whereby family members unwittingly reinforce each other's maladaptive behaviors (Jones, 1980; Patterson, 1975). Consistently paying attention to patients when they complain of pain, for example, will tend to increase the number of complaints, particularly if no attention is paid when patients feel pain-free (Steger & Fordyce, 1982). Walrond-Skinner (1976) notes that often the "identified patient in the family" becomes the focus of attention for every other family member. Even when the patient's behavior is considered negative, family members' attention may provide reinforcement which sustains, rather than punishes, it.

Behavioral intervention in the family takes many forms. Often parents are taught to change the reinforcers they present to children and to apply them in a response contingent manner. The term "response contingent" refers to the presentation of reinforcers only in the presence of a specific stimulus. Behavioral contracts between family members specify desired behaviors and the reinforcers to be given when those behaviors occur. Contingency contracting is often used with couples to enhance reciprocal interaction (Stuart, 1976). Partners list the behaviors they wish each other to exhibit and agree to reinforce those behaviors in a systematic manner. The couple decides upon several behavior-reinforcer pairs, rather than pairing desired behaviors from each other's lists. A response contingent program that pairs behaviors and reinforcers is more likely to be successfully sustained than a contract that simply exchanges desired behaviors and that could easily lead to one partner's refusal to complete the contract if the other fails at any portion of it.

Assertion training, another behavioral method often used with couples, attempts to enhance communication (Lange & Jakubowski, 1976). It is particularly useful with family members who have difficulty expressing strong or negative opinions and emotions. Recently, assertion training has also been used to help impulsive, aggressive individuals express anger more constructively (Rimm & Masters, 1979). Jakubowski-Spector (1973) writes that assertiveness in one family member often precipitates changes in the communication patterns of other family members.

Despite a large number of studies reporting successful behavioral treatment programs for noncompliant individuals (cf. DiMatteo & DiNicola, 1982), the superiority of such programs for enhancing long-term compliance is far from proven. Individual patients often find carrying out such programs difficult. When family members are enlisted, correct and consistent reinforcement of desired behavior often becomes even more difficult to attain (Steger & Fordyce, 1982). Traditionally, behavior therapists have blamed treatment failures on their own inadequate understanding of environmental contingencies and not on the patient's resistance (Wilson & O'Leary, 1981). Cognitive-behavior therapists suggest that the patient's expectations, cognitions, and causal attributions must also be taken into account in treatment failures (Mahoney, 1980). In behavior therapy, however, expression of a desire to comply is generally taken at face value. There is no behavioral or cognitive-behavioral view of the family that emphasizes the uniqueness of the family's role in compliance. Where psychoanalytic family theory may stress the playing out of the individual's conflict with the family over the particular problem of noncompliance, behavioral programs may focus so directly on noncompliance that other family patterns which contribute to the problem are ignored.

Family Systems Theory

Family systems theorists argue that family members are not merely environmental events of the same order as food, sensory stimuli, money, etc., nor are individual members recapitulations of their parents as psychoanalytic family theory suggests. Instead, family systems theory, drawing upon general systems theory and cybernetics, insists that the family is a system of interlocking parts and consists of relationships that are "reciprocal, patterned, and repetitive" (Jones, 1980, p. 43). Any change in one part of the system induces a complementary change in another part but without necessarily changing the rules governing the system.

Four essential concepts in family systems theory are negative feedback, positive feedback, triangulation, and communication. Feedback refers to a process whereby a system changes to maintain homeostasis, or balance. Contrary to common usage, negative feedback does not refer to critical communication but rather to an input from within the system which corrects a deviation and allows the system to remain essentially the same. Positive feedback refers to an input from outside the system that dismantles its current structure and precipitates the formation of a newly balanced one (Foley, 1979).

Negative feedback loops in the family are often found in patterns of triangulation. Bowen (1976) defines triangulation as a set of relationships among three family members that allows two members of the triangle to avoid dealing with a conflict. Foley (1979, p. 462) writes: "Whenever the emotional balance between two people becomes too intense or too distant, a third person or thing can be introduced to restore equilibrium to the system and give it stability." Two common triangular relationships are the mother-father-child group and the father-mother-work pattern.

The degrees of emotional closeness and strength of alliance usually differ between any two dyads of a triangle. The more distance there is between spouses, the closer the child will be to one parent than to the other. If the child attempts to become closer to the formerly distant parent, either the parents' relationship will change, or both parents will alter their relationship to the child and return the triangle to its original degrees of alliance.

Communication, a broad but essential concept in family systems theory, encompasses all interpretable events. Watzlawick, Beavin, and Jackson (1967) argue that "one can not *not* communicate"; verbal responses, nonverbal actions, and silences are all meaningful communications. These theorists contend that every verbal communication not only conveys a content but is also an assertion about what is being said. A husband who tells his wife, "You're always nagging me," is both expressing something about her and asserting the belief and feeling expressed as his own. Statements either imply or specify an instruction for how a particular communication is to be taken. If this husband adds, "I'm only joking," to his first statement, he gives his wife an explicit instruction for how she should take the initial remark. In this case, the explicit instruction overrides the sincerity and negative feeling which the husband's first statement asserted.

In practice, these theoretical distinctions indicate usually unacknowledged aspects of communications that are as much a part of what family members "say" as the content they express. The rules of communication that a family adopts not only govern how and what information can be exchanged but also help define such family patterns as power relationships. If, in the example above, the wife responds by saying, "I don't want to talk about it," she asserts the power to suspend both the conversation and the conflict. If the couple's rules of communication permit the wife to routinely suspend conversation about negative matters in this way, the husband will yield to her statement as an exercising of her dominance. If such a statement breaks their rules, he will take her response as challenging the couple's current power structure.

Communication problems are often rooted in disparities between aspects of communication. These disparities may take on distinctive patterns. The double bind, for example, consists of a "meta-communication" which directly contradicts an overt communication (Bateson, Jackson, Haley, & Weakland, 1956).

A mother scolding her child to "be independent" is giving an inherently contradictory instruction: by becoming independent (the overt communication), the child is merely following her orders (the meta-communication) (Watzlawick, Beavin, & Jackson, 1967). Thus, a person placed in a double bind must choose between two alternatives in a situation where neither choice is satisfactory and leaving the field is not allowed. Haley (1959) notes that in many relationships that employ double-bind communication, one member denies that the double bind exists or that one person controls the other's behavior through its use. Cohen and Wellisch (1978) provide an instance of this tendency in their previously cited case study of a wife who controlled her husband's pain medications while assuring him that he could take them any time.

Ineffective communication patterns such as the double bind present a target for family systems therapists who emphasize the role of communication in creating power relationships. By interfering with such patterns, therapists attempt to precipitate changes in the family's rules of communication. One strategy for interference is to exacerbate the patterns until they fall apart of their own accord (Foley, 1979; Haley, 1976). In principle, homeostasis would then require the adoption of new rules and adjustment of power relationships to sustain them.

Structural family therapy (Minuchin, 1974; Minuchin & Fishman, 1981; Minuchin, Montalvo, & Guerney, 1967) is a particular approach that combines aspects of behavioral and systems orientations. It has been used extensively to treat families in which a chronically ill child is noncompliant or exhibits behavior problems. According to Minuchin (1974), individual family members belong to several subsystems. Each subsystem functions according to a different set of responsibilities and skills, and each gives family members a different level of power over other members. A father may be very powerful as a parent in one subsystem but may be completely cowed by his own parents in another. Each subsystem has boundaries or rules that define its membership, as well as rules governing interactions within it. According to Minuchin et al. (1967), the parents are a subsystem that must operate without interference from grandparents or children in order to function adequately. In maladjusted families, subsystems are often intergenerational, with each parent belonging to a separate subsystem which includes different siblings.

In disengaged families, one member of the parental subsystem sees herself or himself as overwhelmed and controlled by the children or grandparents (Minuchin et al., 1967). In an enmeshed family, one parent—usually the mother—is extremely controlling. The members of an enmeshed family appear overly concerned about each other and do not accept differences between members or subsystems. They strongly resist any attempt to overthrow the control of the one family member who defines the rules of inter-action. Following most family systems theories, structural family therapy asserts that the family maintains an unsuccessful family structure or subsystem by selecting one person as the problem.

Minuchin and his colleagues (Liebman, Minuchin, & Baker, 1974; Minuchin, Rosman, & Baker, 1978) treated families with asthmatic, anorexic, and diabetic children, as well as children with psychosomatic complaints. They found that families with severely asthmatic children were often enmeshed. The entire family life centered around the child's illness. Parents usually assumed that ill children were incapable of handling the physical and emotional stress that accompanied the illness. Parents also continually hovered over the children and observed them for the slightest signs of illness. When an asthma attack occurred, the parents were often unable to treat it adequately, causing both parents and children to panic. The therapists' solutions to the problem placed children in charge of their own treatment. Children were taught breathing exercises, and parents were given specific instructions to follow daily and at the time of an attack. In addition, family therapy sessions helped family members to create natural, more effective subsystems and to differentiate members from one another (Liebman, et al., 1974). Similarly, when dealing with anorexic children in family therapy, Minuchin et al. (1978) changed the parents' focus from the child's refusal to eat as the problem, to their own need to control the child's behavior. The children were encouraged to regulate their own eating through behavior modification procedures, while the family sessions concentrated on the power relationships between the parents, and between the children and parents.

Herz (1980) adds a life-cycle approach to family systems theory. She argues that the impact and meaning of illness and death are different at various times in the life cycle of the family. Each stage of family life demands different roles, responsibilities, and tasks. Illness in old age is considered more natural, even if it is not fully accepted. Early onset of chronic illness interrupts the usual tasks and responsibilities of families. In the family with young children, the death or illness of a spouse forces the surviving or healthy spouse to become sole child-rearer, homemaker, and wage-earner. Chronically ill adolescents may experience a slowing or curtailment of the process of differentiating themselves from the family of origin (Kornfeld & Siegel, 1979). Siblings may resent the attention paid to the ill child, and parents may resent the burdens of caring for the child (cf. Salk et al., 1972). The ill adolescent may rebel against the enmeshment of the family by refusing to comply with medical regimen (Herz, 1980).

As previously mentioned, there have been few empirical studies that relate compliance to family structure. In the studies that have been conducted, the families of compliant patients were more likely to contain a strong parental subsystem, to employ open communication, and to accept differences in family members (Steidl et al., 1980). On the question of the relative efficacy of the various family systems approaches to compliance problems, the literature has been silent.

CASE STUDIES OF FAMILY RELATIONSHIPS AND COMPLIANCE

Chronic illness can trigger changes in every facet of a patient's family life. Shifts in habitual roles are among the most evident and difficult changes. Patients no longer able to work may lose financial security, social or family status, and self-esteem. In traditional families, a husband's inability to work may alter his usual family roles of provider and head of the household. By entering the work force, the wife may share or take over the family's provider role, but the chronically ill husband may be physically incapable of, or unwilling to, assume or share household duties associated with her former role. The wife may feel overburdened and resentful, while the husband may feel his illness denies him a proper role in the family's functioning.

Ill women are generally better able to maintain accustomed

roles than ill men, but the family is more likely to become disorganized when chronic illness impedes the wife-mother's role
than when it affects the father's role (Litman, 1971; 1974). The
wife-mother and family members may both have difficulty with
her adjustment to a receptive, rather than nurturant, role. Not
only must her household duties be relegated, but her role as family
communicator may be compromised or inadequately reassigned.
Single parents who embody all these roles are doubly burdened
by chronic illness. Their children may be called upon to take over
responsibilities usually borne by adults. All patients must find
new ways to occupy time which neither exacerbate the illness
nor conflict with doctors' orders.

From a family systems viewpoint, changes in roles precipitate
changes in power and control within the family. The concepts of
homeostasis, triangulation, enmeshment, and ineffective communication patterns can be used to explain the impact of the family on
compliance problems.

Homeostasis and Role Changes

Noncompliance may maintain the customary roles and tasks
within the family, the level of dominance or dependency of the
ill member, or the family's characteristic methods of resolving
conflict. The disruption or elimination of a patient's usual role
can interfere with compliance even when a conscientious plan
has transferred the duties associated with that role to others.

> Mrs. B., an 84-year-old naturalized American citizen, had a toe removed
> as a result of a diabetic ulcer. She found it very difficult to stay off her
> feet (as ordered) because it had been her lifelong habit to cook large
> meals for her husband and to clean extensively every day. Although her
> daughters regularly performed major cleaning tasks and had arranged
> for daily outside help, Mrs. B. complained that no one could keep house
> as well as she, and that her husband, who was also ill, expected her to
> care for him as she had before.

From a systems viewpoint, although the necessary chores are
performed, the system is unbalanced. Mrs. B. finds it difficult to
comply because compliance deprives her of her usual role vis à
vis her house and her husband. A role reversal, which would main-

tain homeostasis, is not possible because her husband already fills the sick role. Thus, Mrs. B. periodically attempts to reclaim her role by doing forbidden chores she knows others would do at her request.

The family will first attempt to respond to chronic illness as it has responded to other crises in the past. If a submissive or extremely dependent spouse becomes ill, the dominant spouse may manage the other's medication just as he or she might manage finances, household tasks, or other aspects of family life.

> Mrs. M. had always taken charge of bookkeeping and running the family. When her husband had a stroke, she adapted very well to his aphasia, inventing ways to communicate with him. When he developed cancer five years later, she helped him keep track of his medications by putting them in little cups at the beginning of each day, with coded instructions on how many to take and when to take them. In this way, Mr. M., who worried that he hadn't taken his medication, could keep track of it when she wasn't there. Mr. M. was a very compliant patient.

The family member who is the manager is thus able to remain in that role even when the spouse is chronically ill.

Sometimes compliance itself threatens the relationship of the spouses and the homeostasis of the family. To stave off the threat, family members may negotiate the degree of compliance they will accept (Hayes-Bautista, 1976).

> Mr. D., a 57-year old diabetic patient with end-stage renal disease, was so noncompliant with dietary regimen that he endangered his life several times. Mrs. D. did most of the cooking but found it difficult to change her cooking habits. Mr. D. would "scream and yell" at her if she didn't "give him what he wanted." She would feel guilty if she refused to buy or cook the foods he wished. One ineffective compromise was to cook a simple meal but take him to a restaurant for dessert. Mrs. D. would nag her husband about his noncompliance; in turn, he would point out how heavy she and their son were.

For Mrs. D., an ill husband was preferable to a screaming, threatening one. She habitually acquiesed to his wishes and would not consider attempting a behavioral program to extinguish his tantrums. In addition, food was something they could still share, and it therefore served a very important social function for the whole family. Changing rituals surrounding food or eliminating its social and shared function would have required a new activity or ritual that could bring the family together. Mrs. D. reported that she could think of very few activities or interests that the family shared any more.

If the spouse who habitually provided care when others were sick becomes chronically ill, it may be difficult for the other family members to assume the caretaker role. Family members may also presume that the person who usually served as the caretaker (or who is a health professional) will not need the family's help or will adjust to illness easily. Reluctance of the family to deal with the illness itself, or to participate in treatment, may hinder compliance.

> Mrs. S. was a 60-year-old retired nurse who became a hemodialysis patient. She was knowledgeable about different kinds of dialysis treatment and wished to receive home dialysis care. Her husband resisted the option of hemodialysis (which would require his help), stating that, as a nurse, she would be competent to conduct peritoneal dialysis by herself. Mrs. S., who reported that her husband "couldn't deal with illness like I can," eventually chose peritoneal dialysis.

In this case, the decision to have peritoneal dialysis maintained homeostasis in the family by sustaining the distance and independence habitual to their relationship.

Changing the family structure in order to enhance compliance is not always desireable or necessary, particularly if members often solve conflicts by going outside the family.

> Mr. T. was a very active 66-year-old dialysis patient whose wife was a timid, dependent woman. She refused to visit the dialysis clinic because "the contraptions scared" her. She was not a good cook; the couple had arguments about her failure to make meals that complied with Mr. T.'s dialysis diet. Mrs. T. did not want her husband to cook because "he messed up the kitchen." For some years, Mr. T. had eaten at a senior citizen's center four days a week. He decided to review their menus for compatibility with his new diet, rather than ask his wife to change her cooking habits. Mrs. T. accepted his solution amicably, and Mr. T. returned to the center.

In summary, the case studies presented here suggest several ways that medical regimen can upset family homeostasis. Compliance will be harder to achieve when restoring equilibrium requires extensive changes in roles, interaction patterns among family members, and shared family tasks. Among the options for adjusting family roles and tasks to treatment needs, those which diverge least from the current family system are the most likely to be accepted and implemented.

Triangulation

Chronic illness can be incorporated into family patterns of triangulation in two ways: the illness itself may become a "third force" or point in a triangle, or family members may form alliances or subsystems based on their interactions with the ill member. Both these patterns can affect compliance. Minuchin, Rosman, and Baker (1978) suggest that by focusing attention exclusively on a conflict over illness or compliance, the family diffuses a more fundamental conflict between two members.

As Sontag (1978) claims, illness often becomes a metaphor for everything that is wrong in one's personal life or society at large and takes on a character of its own. For families of the chronically ill, the illness can become a scapegoat for the family's problems in dealing with its members. Every unpleasant or trying occurrence is blamed on the illness; every unwanted change of behavior is seen as resulting from the illness rather than from longstanding personality characteristics, understandable events in the environment, or developmental changes in the patient or the family. Most health professionals are familiar with patients who have been "patriarchal, stubborn, and demanding" most of their lives, but whose families regard current instances of such behavior as caused by whatever chronic illness the patient now suffers from.

Attending and adjusting to chronic illness takes much of the family's time and may replace its usual occupations. Some family members arrange their lives around the ill member to the exclusion of other hobbies and activities. They may feel guilty for engaging in enjoyable pursuits when the ill patient is not able to join them.

The "ladies" were three women whose husbands had suffered massive strokes. The patients spent most of their time in a semicomatose state and were deprived of speech, voluntary movement, and any form of communication. For a period of one year, the wives had been coming to the hospital every day to help with the feeding and nursing of their husbands. The wives would trade tasks and chores on the hospital floor and would take care of their friends' husbands when necessary. Overworked nurses welcomed the ladies' help. Their excellent care kept the patients virtually free of bed sores. One of the ladies described her life at the hospital as "a world of its own; it's your whole life." It was emotionally difficult for the ladies to be separated from their husbands. One wife took a full year to decide that she could stay home one day a week without feeling guilty.

Triangulation can be particularly evident in cases involving a condition like chronic pain which interferes with almost every aspect of a patient's life. Chronic pain patients may be unable to work, travel, drive, eat properly, sleep, perform household tasks, relax comfortably, or engage in sexual relations. The behavioral approach to chronic pain contends that pain behavior is often unwittingly reinforced by health professionals and family members (cf. Chapter 4). Such accidental reinforcement may work against the goals of pain management programs designed to maximize the patients' activity levels while minimizing their awareness of, and preoccupation with, pain. A family systems view would add that chronic pain, like all chronic illness, serves some purpose in the family's complex, reciprocal patterns of interaction. Family members may not know what to expect when the patient becomes pain-free. The physical freedom and independence that compliance with pain management treatment fosters may come at the expense of attention, dependency, or the predictability of the family's current behavior and communication patterns.

Mr. E. was a 35-year-old unemployed carpenter who suffered from chronic pain for two years. He was estranged from his family. For the last year, he had been living with Ms. I., an educated woman who supported him financially. To ease his pain, Mr. E. had tried to learn relaxation procedures on his own, before entering an inpatient program for chronic pain management.

In a conjoint counseling session, Ms. I. complained that, although Mr. E. was home all day, he seldom helped with household chores. She felt that he exaggerated the amount of pain he felt when he attempted to do unpleasant tasks. In an individual session, Ms. I. revealed that she was dissatisfied with the relationship but was afraid of telling Mr. E. until he "was ready to handle it." She had the vague feeling that Mr. E. knew she would leave him if he improved.

Without the third force of chronic pain, this couple's relationship could not be sustained. Negative communication was restricted to his condition, and discussion of the fundamental incompatibility Ms. I. perceived between the two of them was postponed. As the patient's stake in the relationship was high, his ultimate success in the treatment program was compromised. In fact, Mr. E. finished the program with only moderate reduction in pain.

Even when illness or treatment are not themselves part of a triangulation pattern, the patient may become part of a family triangle which involves two other family members—especially when the subsystems of the family become intergenerational. By allying themselves with the parents, children may stabilize deteriorating relationships between the spouse and the ill partner. Grown children are often called upon to help their well parent make decisions and care for the ill parent. They may appropriate some parental roles and tasks, such as handling finances. Sometimes the care that the spouse and child must give involves procedures that all parties find uncomfortable or embarrassing, such as giving suppositories.

Taking over the parent's role is especially difficult for adolescents and unmarried young adults. These children may be "parentified" and asked to discipline younger siblings—a duty that the siblings may resent. The ill parent may also resent the child's ascendency. Many ill patients report feeling like children themselves because they are deprived of decision-making roles; many children feel as though they should not have to be parents ahead of their time. In an attempt to reassert authority, the ill parent may rebel against treatment and become particularly demanding, while the child may rebel against giving care.

Mrs. G. was a 64-year-old widow with one leg amputated. She lived with her 13-year-old adopted daughter and 14-year-old adopted son. Two biological children in their thirties lived in other cities. Mr. G. had died suddenly three years before. Mrs. G.'s leg needed to be dressed to prevent ulcers from diabetes. She was severely arthritic, which prevented her from administering her own care. The bulk of care fell to Jane, the 13-year-old daughter. Jane began to be lax in doing the dressing and refused to do household chores. The son was exempt from household tasks because Mrs. G. felt they were women's chores. Although the son had behavior problems in school, Mrs. G. viewed these as less troubling than Jane's problems at home. While the son was sent to live with an older brother, Mrs. G. brought Jane to a children's mental health center for evaluation. She felt that Jane's "unruliness and disobedience" might be evidence of mental illness.

Although not a classical pattern of triangulation, in the case of Mrs. G., noncompliance was related to reliance on an inadequate familial subsystem. Intense demands were placed on one adolescent, while an older sibling was allowed to remain in his appropriate role. Jane became the scapegoat for her mother's resentment of the illness and drew attention away from the son's problems.

When young married adults become chronically ill, their parents may behave as if the illness were an opportunity to regain control over their children. A triangle consisting of the parent, child, and the child's spouse may occur, especially if there was originally conflict between the young couple or between the parent and the child's spouse. The patient is often caught between two subsystems, but by focusing on the illness, family members in the triangle deflect the nature of the original conflict between subsystems.

Mr. F. was a 22-year-old serviceman who became a quadraplegic as a result of a freak accident. He was married to a servicewoman, and they had a one-year-old child who resided with the wife's parents. The marriage had been very stormy, and Mr. F.'s family disliked his wife. Mr. F.'s mother was given power of attorney, which included receiving and controlling his paychecks. The mother felt that the wife's decision to stay in the service indicated a lack of love. The wife accused the mother of plotting against her and ruining her marriage. Neither wife nor mother would confront each other directly but would tell the patient about their misgivings, implying that the patient would have to make a choice between them. Mr. F. became very depressed, stating that he had no control over his body nor his life and that he was little more than a baby. He stopped going to rehabilitation therapies and made little progress. Eventually he went home with his mother but made plans to hire an aide to help with his care.

Occasionally, the illness of the parent may realign already triangulated families into more effective subsystems. Spouses may be forced to work together, rather than to focus on, or fight through, the children. Mrs. M., the efficient manager described earlier, had a very child-centered family. When her husband became terminally ill, she decided to ask her grown children to move out of the house. When they did, she reported that her relationship with both her husband and children improved. She argued with her husband and children less, and her husband seemed to complain of pain less.

Enmeshment and Communication Patterns

As mentioned earlier, Minuchin, Rosman, and Baker (1978) contend that many families with chronically ill members tend to be enmeshed. Enmeshed families show little tolerance for individuation and independence of members, although they ostensibly wish that the members would become more independent. The chronically ill member is a focal point around whom the other members rally, and through whom members argue. In enmeshed families, the members tend to take over the care of the patient. For the patient, noncompliance becomes a way of asserting control over oneself and other family members. Enmeshed family members sometimes view the noncompliance of the patient as a personal failure or as a rejection of their love.

> Mrs. R. was a 63-year-old widow with end-stage renal disease, who was about to begin dialysis. She also had diabetes and was noncompliant with her restricted diet. She had three children, two of whom had several toddlers. One daughter lived with Mrs. R. in a small apartment. This daughter "got sick at the sight of blood" and was not able to help her mother take insulin or other medications. A second daughter, Mary, had learned to walk despite having polio as a child. The son remained detached from his mother's medical problems. Mary was seen as the manager by her siblings, who felt that Mary was too hard on Mrs. R. when she was noncompliant. Mary felt that her mother was not only noncompliant but that she was wasting her life by spending time reading novels and watching TV. She resented her sister's refusal to help and was highly critical of the whole family's handling of Mrs. R.'s illness. The siblings felt that Mary was taking just as much advantage of Mrs. R. as they were, by having her babysit regularly. Mary felt that it was her duty to stand by her mother and help her, "just as she helped me when I had polio." Mrs. R. found Mary to be too "bossy."

In the case of Mrs. R., the family was interdependent, but members did not get along. The children were either overly involved in the patient's life, or they were not involved at all. One daughter saw her mother's situation as similar to one she experienced as a child and quite consciously wanted to mother her own mother. At the same time, she refused to allow her mother freedom of choice and demanded that her siblings view the problem exactly as she herself viewed it. The mother found herself caught in the middle: she wanted help from the children who would not give it and wanted to refuse help from the child who offered it. In an effort to "live the way I want to," she chose noncompliance.

When both spouses are ill, as is often the case with elderly couples, neither spouse may be able to adequately fulfill roles or give proper attention to compliance with medical regimen. They may bicker about each other's health, using a "symmetrical" communication pattern (Watzlawick, Beavin, & Jackson, 1967) in which each tries to outdo the other in number of complaints or in proving that the other is taking inadequate care of himself or herself.

> Mr. O., a 77-year-old retired Army officer with end-stage renal disease, had been receiving dialysis for four months. Mrs. O. was also ill. She complained that her husband's personality had changed since beginning dialysis. In turn, Mr. O. complained that his wife was forgetful and suspicious of him and the neighbors. Mrs. O. managed to prepare tasty meals that followed the strict diet dictated for kidney patients but shopping for the necessary ingredients often took her hours. She would return home very tired. Mr. O. apparently sneaked liquids forbidden in the diet when she was gone. He was genuinely concerned about his wife's health but felt too tired and too incompetent to help her shop or to do chores around the house. She responded by arguing that if he stuck to his diet he would feel better and could then help her. Mr. O. considered such remarks to be nagging.

The wife was given the opportunity to meet weekly with professional staff to discuss her complaints. Although the patient (who correctly viewed his condition as terminal) did not become more compliant, the wife found that she could limit her nagging because of the sessions, and the couple reported that they bickered less.

The case studies presented here were selected because they clearly illustrated common family problems. Obviously, many noncompliant families maintain maladaptive family systems with problems that cannot be defined by a single concept. The final case example, presented below, describes a troubled family with a variety of conflicts that hinder compliance.

> Mr. P. was a 55-year-old dialysis patient who had been on home dialysis for the past 13 years. Mrs. P. became ill and felt unable to help her husband with home dialysis. Mr. P. began going to the hospital for dialysis. He became very depressed, which was unusual for him, and began to have problems following his diet. Although her health improved, Mrs. P. was reluctant to admit she was well enough to resume home dialysis assistance.
>
> Discussion with the couple revealed that Mr. P. had plans to move back to his home town in a rural area out of state. The family kept putting off the move, although they had bought a house, and one son had already moved. Without directly vetoing the move, Mrs. P. would raise indirect objections to it. Mr. P. was also having second thoughts which he would not admit to his spouse.
>
> Both Mr. and Mrs. P. began to dredge up the past. Several years before, Mrs. P. discovered that her husband was having a long-term affair with another woman. Mrs. P. was still very angry with him but felt she could not express her anger. She was afraid that her husband's family in the new town might find out about this now ended affair and judge her an unfit wife, or that if her husband started another affair in the new town "everyone would know about it."

In this family, the spouses had dealt with chronic illness by adjusting roles and by cooperating in treatment. However, communication about their relationship and the role illness played in holding them together was never direct. Alternating cycles of illness would temporarily focus attention on whichever spouse felt overburdened or left out. An ill wife could not reasonably be expected to take care of her husband, nor could two ill people be expected to move. Similarly, an ill, depressed husband would foster pity on the part of the wife rather than anger. Compliance played only a minor and shifting part in the trenchancy of the interpersonal patterns developed by the couple for handling stress and conflict.

INTERVENTION

Intervention with families to enhance compliance takes three major forms: family support groups, family or couples therapy, and behavioral training programs. Some families may participate in all three kinds of programs. It is clear that no single theoretical formulation or therapeutic technique will be sufficient to solve all compliance problems. In general, the most effective individual psychotherapeutic treatment attempts to directly modify emotional, behavioral, and cognitive aspects of problems, rather than centering on only one of these elements (Mahoney, 1980). By extension, interventions with families that are aimed at enhancing compliance must also address these three components. Today, most health practitioners are only intuitively aware of the potential impact of the family on compliance. At the present time, no controlled research for comparing the relative efficacy of different familial interventions for compliance exists. Therefore, when faced with incorporating family members into programs designed to enhance compliance, doctors, psychologists, occupational therapists, and other health practitioners are forced to design remedies on the wing. Ideally, researchers and practitioners concerned with families and compliance must formulate a well-integrated theoretical framework leading to specific and replicable treatment techniques amenable to empirical research.

REFERENCES

Aho, W. R. Relationship of wives' preventive health orientation to their beliefs about heart disease in husbands. *Public Health Reports*, *92*(1), 65-71, 1977.

Baric, L. Conjugal roles as indicators of family influence on health directed action. *International Journal of Health Education*, *13*, 58-65, 1970.

Bateson, G., Jackson, D. D., Haley, J., & Weakland, J. Toward a theory of schizophrenia. *Behavior Science*, *1*, 251-264, 1956.

Becker, M. H., & Green, L. W. A family approach to compliance with medical treatment—A selective review of the literature. *International Journal of Health Education*, *18*, 1-11, 1975.

Becker, M. H., Kaback, M. M., Rosenstock, I. M., & Ruth, M. V. Some influences on public participation in a genetic screening program. *Journal of Community Health*, *1*, 3-14, 1975.

Becker, M. H., & Maiman, L. A. Strategies for enhancing patient compliance. *Journal of Community Health*, *6*, 113-135, 1980.

Bowen, M. Theory in the practice of psychotherapy. In P. Guerin (Ed.), *Family therapy: Theory and practice*. New York: Gardner Press, 42-90, 1976.

Carter, E. A., & McGoldrick, M. *The family life cycle: A framework for family therapy.* New York: Gardner Press, 1980.

Cohen, P., Dizenhuz, I. M., & Winget, C. Family adaptation to terminal illness and death of a parent. *Social Casework, 58*(4), 223–228, 1977.

Cohen, M. M., & Wellisch, D. K. Living in limbo: Psychosocial intervention in families with a cancer patient. *American Journal of Psychotherapy, 32*(4), 561–571, 1978.

Dapitch-Miura, E., & Hovell, M. F. Contingency management of adherence to a complex medical regimen in an elderly heart patient. *Behavior Therapy, 10*(2), 193–201, 1979.

Diamond, M. D., Weiss, A. J., & Grynbaum, B. The unmotivated patient. *Archives of Physical Medicine and Rehabilitation, 49,* 281–284, 1968.

DiMatteo, M. R., & DiNicola, D. D. *Achieving patient compliance: The psychology of the medical practitioner's role.* New York: Pergamon Press, 1982.

DiMatteo, M. R., & Hays, R. Social support and serious illness. In B. Gottlieb (Ed.), *Social networks and social support.* Beverly Hills, CA: Sage Publications, 117–148, 1981.

Foley, V. Family therapy. In R. Corsini (Ed.), *Current psychotherapies* (2nd edition). Itasca, IL: F. E. Peacock, 1979.

Framo, J. Family of origin as a therapeutic resource for adults in marital and family therapy: You can and should go home again. *Family Process, 15,* 193–210, 1976.

Green, L. W., Levine, D. M., & Wolle, J. Development of randomized patient education experiments with urban poor hypertensives. *Patient Counselling and Health Education, 1,* 106–111, 1979.

Gurman, A. S., & Kniskern, D. P. *Handbook of family therapy.* New York: Brunner/Mazel, 1981.

Haley, J. An interactional description of schizophrenia. *Psychiatry, 22,* 321–332, 1959.

Haley, J. *Problem solving therapy.* San Francisco: Jossey-Bass, 1976.

Hayes-Bautista, D. E. Modifying the treatment: Patient compliance, patient control, and medical care. *Social Science and Medicine, 10,* 233–238, 1976.

Heinzelmann, F., & Bagley, R. W. Response to physical activity programs and their effects on health behavior. *Public Health Reports, 85,* 905–911, 1970.

Herz, F. The impact of death and serious illness on the family life cycle. In E. A. Carter & M. McGoldrick, *The family life cycle: A framework for family therapy.* New York: Gardner Press, 1980.

Jakubowski-Spector, P. *An introduction to assertive training procedures for women.* Washington, DC: American Personnel and Guidance Association, 1973.

Jones, S. L. *Family therapy: A comparison of approaches.* Bowie, MD: Robert J. Brady Co., 1980.

Karoly, P. Operant methods. In F. Kanfer & A. Goldstein, *Helping people change.* London: Pergamon, 1975.

Kornfeld, M. S., & Siegel, I. M. Parental group therapy in the management of fatal childhood disease. *Health and Social Work, 4*(3), 99–118, 1979.

Lange, A., & Jakubowski, P. *Responsible assertive behavior: Cognitive-behavioral procedures for trainers.* Champaign, IL: Research Press, 1976.

Liberman, R. Behavioral approaches to family and couple therapy. In G. D. Erickson & T. P. Hogan (Eds.), *Family therapy: An introduction to theory and technique.* Monterey, CA: Brooks/Cole, 120–134, 1972.

Liebman, R., Minuchin, S., & Baker, L. The use of structural family therapy in the treatment of intractable asthma. *American Journal of Psychiatry, 131,* 535–540, 1974.

Litman, T. J. Health care and the family: A three generational analysis. *Medical Care, 9,* 67–81, 1971.

Litman, T. J. The family as basic unit in health and medical care: A social behavioral overview. *Social Science and Medicine, 8,* 495–519, 1974.

Litman, T. J., & Venters, M. Research on health care and the family: A methodological overview. *Social Science and Medicine, 13A,* 379–385, 1979.

MacElveen, P. M. Cooperative triad in hemodialysis care and patient outcomes. *Communicating Nursing Research, 5,* 134–147, 1972.

Mahoney, M. J. *Abnormal psychology: Perspectives in human variance.* New York: Harper & Row, 1980.

Minuchin, S. *Families and family therapy.* Cambridge, MA: Harvard University Press, 1974.

Minuchin, S., & Fishman, H. C. *Family therapy techniques.* Cambridge, MA: Harvard University Press, 1981.

Minuchin, S., Montalvo, B., & Guerney, B. *Families of the slums: An exploration of their structure and treatment.* New York: Basic Books, 1967.

Minuchin, S., Rosman, B. L., & Baker, L. *Psychosomatic families.* Cambridge, MA: Harvard University Press, 1978.

Muller, C. Income and the receipt of medical care. *American Journal of Public Health, 55,* 510–521, 1965.

Oakes, T. W. Family expectations and arthritis patient compliance to a hand resting splint regimen. *Journal of Chronic Disease, 22,* 757–764, 1970.

O'Brien, M. D. Role relations and social work needs of married diabetics. *Dissertation Abstracts International, 39*(11-A), 6973, 1979.

Osterweis, M., Bush, P. J., & Zuckerman, A. E. Family context as a predictor of individual medicine use. *Social Science and Medicine, 13A,* 287–291, 1979.

Patterson, G. *Families: Applications of social learning to family life.* Champaign, IL: Research Press, 1975.

Rimm, D. C., & Masters, J. C. *Behavior therapy: Techniques and empirical findings* (2nd edition). New York: Academic Press, 1979.

Salk, L., Hilgartner, M., & Granich, B. The psychosocial impact of hemophilia on the patient and his family. *Social Science and Medicine, 6,* 491–505, 1972.

Slivkin, S. E. Death and living: A family therapy approach. *American Journal of Psychoanalysis, 37*(4), 317–323, 1977.

Sontag, S. *Illness as metaphor.* New York: Farrar, Straus, and Giroux, 1978.

Steger, J., & Fordyce, W. Behavioral health care in the management of pain. In T. Millon, C. Green, & R. Meagher, *Handbook of clinical health psychology.* New York: Plenum Press, 1982.

Steidl, J. H., Finkelstein, F. O., Wexler, J. P., Feigenbaum, H., Kitsen, J., Kliger, A. S., & Quinlan, D. M. Medical condition, adherence to treatment regimens, and family functioning. *Archives of General Psychiatry, 37*, 1025–1027, 1980.

Stuart, R. B. An operant interpersonal program for couples. In D. H. L. Olson (Ed.), *Treating relationships*. Lake Mills, IA: Graphic, 1976.

Tucker, M. Effect of heavy medical expenditures on low income families, incidence and impact. *Public Health Reports, 85*, 419–425, 1970.

Vogel, E. F., & Bell, N. W. The emotionally disturbed child as the family scapegoat. In N. W. Bell & E. F. Vogel (Eds.), *A modern introduction to the family*. New York: Free Press, 1968.

Walrond-Skinner, S. W. *Family therapy: The treatment of natural systems*. London: Routledge and Kegan Paul, 1976.

Watzlawick, P., Beavin, J. H., & Jackson, D. D. *Pragmatics of human communication*. New York: W. W. Norton, 1967.

Weber, W. C. Families cope with stress: A study of family strengths in families where a spouse had end-stage renal disease. *Dissertation Abstracts International, 41*(11-A), 4579–4580, 1981.

Whitehead, M. C. Psychological factors affecting compliance to a medical treatment program: A study of mother participation in home infusion therapy for hemophiliacs. *Dissertation Abstracts International, 42*(5-B), 2036, 1981.

Wilson, G. T., & O'Leary, K. D. *Principles of behavior therapy*. Englewood Cliffs, NJ: Prentice-Hall, 1981.

Wingert, W. A., Larson, W., Friedman, D. B. The influence of familial organization on the utilization of pediatric emergency services. *Pediatrics, 42*, 743, 1968.

7

The Special Case of Compliance in the Elderly

Phyllis L. Amaral

Rehabilitative regimens depend heavily on patient compliance. The present chapter deals with how compliance can be enhanced in older adults—a population whose health profile makes them prime targets for rehabilitative rather than acute intervention. Since older adults have many more rehabilitative needs than any other age group, their unique characteristics should be considered when compliance strategies are devised.

This chapter first sets out the particular health and compliance issues facing older people. Then, the physical, environmental, and psychological barriers to compliance for the older adult will be discussed, based on both social gerontological and health care literatures. Those barriers derived from the social gerontological literature have not generally been addressed in relation to compliance.

Research on strategies to enhance compliance in older adults will be explored and briefly summarized. This section will illustrate the multidimensional nature of the problems associated with compliance. Finally, a model of geriatric health care will be presented that deals with the range of barriers to compliance in the older adult. This model offers a multifaceted approach to potential barriers without placing unrealistic demands on the physician-patient relationship.

The author gratefully acknowledges the assistance of Debra Cherry, LaDonna Ringering, Raphe Sonenshein, and Steven Zarit in the development of this chapter.

THE SCOPE OF THE PROBLEM

Health Problems of the Older Adult

Individuals become increasingly vulnerable to illness and dependent on health care services as they age. For example, in 1973, persons 65 years or older (approximately 10 percent of the population) accounted for 28 percent of the 80 billion dollar bill for personal health care in the United States (Shanas & Maddox, 1976). According to the United States Department of Health, Education and Welfare, National Center for Health Statistics (1971),

> The lives of millions of older Americans are affected daily by illness or impairments, for chronic health problems increase sharply with age. Indeed, chronic diseases might well be called "companions of the aged." The statistics are striking: 85 percent of those 65 and over living outside institutions—15 million people—have at least one chronic condition, and about half of those individuals suffer some limitation of activity because of chronic conditions. (p. 17)

What kinds of chronic conditions are prevalent among the elderly? Several studies have demonstrated that blood pressure, particularly systolic pressure, is higher in older persons than younger persons (Bierman & Brody, 1980). In fact, prevalence rates for hypertension are approximately 26 percent and 46 percent for white men and women, respectively. Rates for black older adults are significantly higher (54 percent for men; 65 percent for women) with less discrepancy (U.S. Department of Health, Education and Welfare, National Center for Health Statistics, 1971). Heart disease is also strongly age-related. At ages 45—64, about one-sixth of white men and women and one-third of black men and women have heart disease. Over the age of 65, these rates increase to one-third and about two-fifths of white men and women, respectively. Again, prevalence rates are much higher for older black persons. Definite heart disease is found in about one-half of the black women and fully 70 percent of the black males over 65 years of age.

Another strongly age-related disease is diabetes, found in 3 percent of the men and 6 percent of the women over 65. According to Bierman and Brody (1980), its role as a cause of disability—blindness, kidney failure, neurological problems, arteriosclerosis of the coronary and leg vessels—and of early death has been previously underestimated.

Osteoarthritic degenerative joint disease primarily affects joint cartilage and can cause significant impairment. Estimates suggest that approximately 60 percent of the elderly suffer this affliction (Bierman & Brody, 1980). Osteoporosis—a skeletal disorder whereby bone is lost with age so that the body cannot easily handle wear and tear—significantly increases the older person's susceptibility to bone fractures. Osteoporosis is four times more common in women. Approximately 6.3 million people suffer problems related to weakened vertebrae. Surgery for hip fracture is the third most common procedure in people over 65. According to Bierman and Brody (1980), "The high disability and death rates that ensue are out of proportion to the severity of the trauma; they reflect the difficulties of major surgery followed by prolonged immobilization and loss of independence" (p. 17).

Specific types of cancer—breast cancer, cancer of the large intestine, and chronic lymphatic leukemia—occur with high frequency in the elderly relative to other age groups. For example, 50 percent of all breast cancers are diagnosed at age 60 or older. The incidence of cancer rises sharply as the population ages. According to Seidman, Silverberg, & Bodden (1978), data indicate that the probability of developing cancer between the ages of 20 and 40 is approximately 1 percent for men and 1.5 percent for women. Between ages 65 and 85, probabilities increase to approximately 17 percent for women and 23 percent for men. More than one-half of all cancers occur in people over the age of 65 (Kennedy, undated).

Other chronic problems with which the elderly must contend can include parkinsonism, respiratory disease, altered response to infection, cerebrovascular disease, dementia, and sensory losses. Each of these chronic—sometimes fatal—diseases bring along a unique set of challenges to face. In general, however, one can predict psychological and behavioral reactions to illness that transcend the specifics of the illness. Indeed, Bierman and Brody (1980) have asserted that "the expected symptoms of anxiety and depression accompanying illness are so common that they have indeed become 'diagnoses' " (p. 24).

Restricted mobility and constraints on daily routine can also be expected. In fact, approximately two-fifths of persons 65 years and over suffer some limitation in activity because of chronic conditions, according to the U.S. Department of Health, Education and Welfare (1971). In a more recent survey of older persons in Chicago, between 40 and 65 percent of the sample groups admitted to having disabilities or impairments that limited their activities (Bild & Havighurst, 1976). However, Kovar (1977) reported that 82 percent of noninstitutionalized elderly nationwide reported no limitation in mobility and that they did not need the help of a person or device to get around. Apparently estimates of disability among the aged vary considerably depending upon the constraints of the question to which older people responded.

In sum, physical illnesses—many of which require active and aggressive rehabilitation regimens—appear with extraordinary frequency and variety in older adults. Strategies to improve compliance then are particularly important to reduce the physical hazards and improve the quality of life associated with growing old.

Compliance

Roughly speaking, older persons resemble the broader population with respect to their degree of compliance with medication. For example, Sackett and Snow (1979) surveyed a variety of studies reporting compliance rates with different long-term medication regimens for different illnesses and different settings and found a tendency for those rates to converge around 50 percent. Similarly, a sample of the literature concerning adherence to prescription medication regimens for older adults reported compliance rates ranging from 38 percent to 57 percent with an average rate of roughly 45 percent (Cooper, Love, & Raffoul, 1982; Curtis, 1961; Hemminki & Heikkilä, 1975; Neely & Patrick, 1968; Schwartz, Wang, Zeitz, & Goss, 1962). The duration for which the drug was prescribed (long-term versus short-term) is unclear in some of these studies, however, so the rates are not entirely comparable. Sackett and Snow (1979) also report that compliance with appointment-keeping for all adults in a variety of settings is approximately 50 percent when the appointment is suggested by a health professional and increases to approximately 75 percent when the patient initiates the appointment. With regard to this type of medical service, older persons may be more compliant. This is suggested by an investigation (Brand & Smith, 1974) of 114 chronically ill elderly patients six months after discharge from a general hospital. Only about 14 percent noncompliance was evidenced with respect to medical appointments with a much higher noncompliance rate to outpatient department appointments (24 percent) than to physician office visits (9 percent). Again, compliance rates cited for the general adult population may not be entirely comparable to those cited for older adults since the former estimate included several investigations of compliance to appointment keeping for prevention (e.g., breast cancer screening, appointment following hypertension screening). Reasons for physician-suggested follow-ups in the investigation of chronically ill elderly persons were not specified but presumably were relatively serious given their close proximity to hospital discharge.

Brand and Smith (1974) presented other compliance rates that offer additional perspective on the chronically ill elderly. Apparently, suggestions for nursing services (e.g., bedside care, injections) met with widespread approval and yielded a compliance rate of 92 percent. Conversely, suggestions for rehabilitation services (e.g., speech therapy, physical therapy) were complied with only 50 percent of the time. Interestingly, this investigation reported compliance with oral medication requirements by 87 percent—the best drug compliance rate reported. However, criteria for compliance were not specified. Finally, recommended changes in diet and smoking or alcohol consumption met with 55 percent and 57 percent compliance rates, respectively.

BARRIERS

The previous section detailed the wide variety of health problems facing older people—problems that require substantial compliance with rehabilitative regimens.

This section explores the physical, environmental, and psychological barriers to compliance that characterize the elderly population. Individual older adults may exhibit none of the problems described below. On the other hand, only by understanding these barriers can we begin to design appropriate strategies to enhance compliance among those elderly they unduly restrict.

Physical Barriers

Vision

According to the National Center for Health Statistics (1971) 7 out of 8 persons 45 years and older wear glasses or contact lenses all or part time, compared with 3 out of 10 persons 18-24 years old. In fact, demographic research has shown that age is the single best predictor of visual impairment (Hatfield, 1973). At 65 years of age and older, 75 percent of women and 67 percent of men have at least a mild vision deficit (20/30 or worse) even with correction. Mild to moderate vision deficits have little practical relevance to compliance behavior. However, severe vision impairments, which also increase with age, can seriously impede compliance.

Genensky and Zarit (in press) have provided age-wise distributions of populations with severe vision loss. According to their estimates, approximately 54 percent of partially sighted persons—1,044,500 individuals—are estimated to be at least 65 years old. (In general terms, most partially sighted persons are unable to read newspaper column type at normal reading distances, even with the help of conventional eyeglasses, and have difficulty recognizing familiar faces unless they are very close.) In addition to this group of people, 46 percent of the functionally blind population—persons who have, at most, light projection—are also 65 years or older.

There are far more older adults who are partially sighted than are functionally blind. Many of the vision conditions common in this age group—glaucoma, macular degeneration, cataracts—leave the individual with useable vision than can be enhanced with appropriate visual aids. However, less than one percent of the eye care facilities nationwide provide their patients with a program of vision enhancement through the use of specialized optical and nonoptical aids and services.

For older adults with a severe vision impairment, proper management of prescription medication can become a near impossibility. A 64-year-old patient at a low vision clinic serves as an illustrative case:

> Beside coping with increasingly poor vision over the past four years, this patient—who has no nearby relatives—also is faced with a host of other physical problems. When he came to the attention of the vision clinic, he had at least 10 prescription medications in his possession and was taking none of them. Unable to read his own writing or the labels on each bottle, the patient had long forgotten the prescribed regimens. Additionally, he could not differentiate one medicine from another nor could he read the expiration date on any of his p.r.n. (as needed) medications. The patient was fearful that his physical condition would deteriorate and understandably frustrated that health care seemed out of his control.

As illustrated in this case, the implications of low vision for compliance behavior are clear. Well over one million older adults lack a critical element in adhering to rehabilitation regimens—adequate vision. Many do not receive the help they need to compensate for their visual impairment. Even those older adults who do have access to low vision aids will, in all likelihood, continue to have difficulty reading the small type on prescription labels, especially if the print is light, and will generally have difficulty reading all printed materials where the contrast is poor (e.g., light copies of instructions, mimeographed protocols or instructions).

Hearing

Approximately 30 percent of individuals 65–79 have "significant impairment of hearing in the frequencies essential in the range associated with normal speech" (Shanas & Maddox, 1976). Decker (1974) has reported that 70 percent of the patients 50 years and older who were treated in the rehabilitation department of a large metropolitan hospital had hearing losses sufficient to prevent them from interacting in a satisfactory manner with those around them. Apparently, in this sample, hearing aids were greatly underutilized, and Decker (1974) listed two primary reasons for underuse: cost of high quality hearing aids and lack of understanding about the potential of hearing aids. Additionally, even when hearing losses are correctible by hearing aids, the aid may be difficult to use in certain situations (e.g., when there is substantial background noise). Indeed, the National Center for Health Statistics data (1971) indicate that among persons 45 years and over with a hearing loss in both ears, only about 20 percent use a hearing aid.

Again, the implications for compliance are clear. Critical communications can be missed by the patient with a hearing deficit. An important extension of this line of thought is found in a study of the relationship between mild hearing losses and cognitive functioning in older individuals whose hearing was essentially within normal limits (Granick, Klehan, & Weiss, 1976). Even in the face of relatively normal aural function, substantial associations between hearing losses on verbal intelligence tests (especially those tests involving use of stored information, grasp of abstract relationships, definition of concepts) were identified. At this point, the data are merely suggestive, but as the authors conclude, it does lead to questions about how hearing acuity interacts with learning. A possible future consideration will concern better ways in which to communicate a rehabilitative protocol such that comprehension is enhanced, requisite learning is assured, and the older adult is able to completely carry out necessary therapeutic regimens.

Environmental Barriers

Over and above physical difficulties, there are several practical impediments to compliance. Because these barriers are already widely recognized as dilemmas of the elderly, they will only be given brief attention here.

Income

Financial status is a major source of concern to most older adults. Even with existing supplemental programs (e.g., Social Security), older persons do not fare well economically. For example, 14 percent of all noninstitutionalized individuals over the age of 65 subsist below the poverty level in the United States. An additional 25 percent or 5 million older Americans live just above the poverty line (the Federal Council on Aging, 1981). Brand, Smith, and Brand (1977) have identified cost as a significant factor in compliance. They stated that elderly people who are chronically ill and patients in lower socioeconomic groups were especially affected by the cost of prescription medication. More generally, estimates of Medicare coverage (Lohmann, 1981; Shomaker, 1982) indicate that this program (in three different years) picked up less than 50 percent of personal health costs of old and poor individuals. Many vital needs—especially in a population with high incidence of chronic illness—are deemed primary prevention and are left unpaid. Such needs include most types of glasses, hearing aids, various prescriptions, routine physical examinations, and dental care (Shomaker, 1982).

Transportation

Transportation needs differ drastically depending on geographical area, living situation, and ability to drive. However, sensory losses, multiple chronic illnesses (e.g., heart disease and rheumatoid arthritis), and no available immediate family can sorely hamper the older adult's ability to keep physician appointments, to adhere to a rehabilitation regimen that requires frequent trips to a health provider (e.g., physical therapy), or even to reach a pharmacy to obtain prescription medications.

For example, at our low vision rehabilitation clinic that serves primarily older adults (approximately 70 percent are age 60 or over), 63 percent reported problems with bus transportation (Center for the Partially Sighted, 1980). Additionally, one-third of our patient population lives alone, making it difficult to arrange transportation with family or friends. While characteristics of the patient population served may inflate the number of individuals experiencing transportation problems, this example serves to illustrate how routine aspects of living (getting around in the community) can sabotage the older adult's health care needs.

Social Isolation

Social isolation can have serious repercussions for the older adult. Although not indicative of a mental disorder, the response to social isolation resembles the effects of mental disorders, including cognitive impairment and poor social adjustment. Approximately 30 percent of persons over the age of 65 live alone. An extraordinary sex difference is present with only 15 percent of elderly men and nearly 41 percent of elderly women living alone. Living alone does not always imply isolation. For example, approximately 80 percent of persons over 65 have at least one surviving child and about 75 percent of those adults with children saw them within the last week (Federal Council on the Aging, 1981).

However, even in the best of situations, where parent and child have an easy, mutually enjoyable relationship, this contact may not compensate for a lost spouse or a dwindling social network. Individuals who would have been classified as loners in their earlier years are typically comfortable with that lifestyle in later years (Lowenthal & Robinson, 1976). For the many older people characterized by numerous friendships and activities throughout their lives, social curtailment, if it occurs, can be devastating.

In practical terms, the repercussions of social isolation can seriously impede crucial doctor–patient communication. Imagine a situation in which an elderly person approaches a health care professional after having little contact with other individuals—except perhaps an occasional friend or family member—for a prolonged period of time. Most likely, the older person's social skills would be rusty, thus altering the nature of conversation by appearing abrupt, tentative, or confused. Moreover, the individual might have definite problems framing questions and may not be able to respond with necessary information in the allotted time. Consequently, compliance is sabotaged because the information on which the rehabilitation protocol is based is sketchy, incomplete, and potentially inaccurate.

Inadequate Therapeutic Regimens

This catch-all category includes several separate issues that potentially sabotage the older adult's ability or willingness to comply. A few examples will be summarized below:

Over-Prescription. Due in part to the increased prevalence of illness with old age, medication plays a large role in the older adult's life. While older adults comprise only 10 percent of the population in the United States, they consume about 25 percent of the prescription drugs and about the same proportion of non-prescription drugs (Lindsay, 1981; Lofholm, 1974). Much has been written about the problems of polypharmacy and drug inter-action in this age group. We are beginning to consider age-asso-ciated physiological changes in absorption, metabolism, liver and renal function, etc., that make older adults particularly vulnerable to drug interactions and drug side effects (Ouslander, 1981; Weg, 1974). However, adverse drug reactions continue to plague the older adult population. For example, Lindsay (1981) summarized data indicating that 24 percent of a group of hospitalized patients 80 years or older demonstrated adverse drug reactions in contrast with 12 percent of those patients between the ages of 40–50. Additionally, another study surveyed indicated that of the three percent admission rate for adverse drug reactions to the University of Florida Hospital, 40 percent were over the age of 60. Finally, Butler (1976) has cited data from the American College of Neuro-psychopharmacology estimating that three to six percent of a mixed psychiatric population may develop tardive dyskinesia and that chronic older patients have a 20 percent rate.

In an article dealing with the overuse of tranquilizers, Butler (1976) asserts, "Often drugs represent the only form of treatment given to older persons. An overall treatment plan that includes attention to diet, physical and social activities, psychotherapy and correction of living problems may be totally ignored" (p. 186). Perhaps our attitudes toward older adults—discussed more fully in the following section—lead to an overreliance on medication in the face of other viable treatment protocols.

One example of the tendency to view medication as the treat-ment of choice was presented by a colleague:

> A 68-year-old woman, along with her husband, had settled in a retire-ment community when they sold their family business. Although happy with the move, she was experiencing some added stress stemming from her efforts to adjust to her new life. Always an energetic, anxious person, this woman complained of a sleep disturbance at one of her annual physicals. Due to the presence of this symptom, which, in combination with other symptoms can indicate depression, and the presence of anxiety (which was long-standing), the patient was given a combination antianxiety, antidepressent medication. The patient ignored directions

printed on the label to take the medication daily and rather used it sporadically when she had difficulty sleeping. She was not satisfied with the results and discontinued it when she discovered the purpose of the drug.

The main issue in this case is not whether the drug prescribed was the appropriate drug but whether any prescription was in order at all. When questioned about her expectations, the patient stated that she wanted something she could take occasionally if she experienced sleeping difficulties. The patient was surprised when she learned more about the medication she was taking because she considered herself neither depressed nor uncomfortably anxious. Moreover, she did not want any medication she would have to take daily. In her mind, she had been given a solution to the wrong problem. Had the patient been privy to her doctor's logic, she may have agreed to the prescribed drug regimen. Or, she would have rejected the drug outright and perhaps forced a discussion of other alternatives. As the situation was framed, she tried to alter the regimen to suit her needs without the benefits of her physician's expertise—resulting in drug misuse.

Pfeiffer (1980) has supplied reasons for the emphasis on and misuse of medication that suggest the need for a future concentration on both public and professional education. First, he maintains that physicians are generally not taught to alter drastically drug doses consistent with age-related physiological changes. On the other hand, Pfeiffer points to the expectation of older adults to receive medication for all their ailments and suggests that the pressure on the physicians to prescribe is high. Finally, Pfeiffer cites television advertising as a culprit, pointing out that implicit in the advertising is the suggestion that medication will solve a wide variety of psychosocial problems (e.g., loneliness) associated with aging or other problems of daily living that may well be best handled through counseling or social interaction.

Older adults tend to make more medication errors as the number of their medications increases (Curtis, 1961; Hulka, Cassei, Kupper, & Burdette, 1976; Neely & Patrick, 1968). Other factors associated with noncompliance in older samples include household composition (Schwartz et al., 1962); cost (Brand et al., 1977); inability to handle containers and lack of patient education

(Atkinson et al., 1977); among others. Hemminki and Heikkila (1975) have suggested that the type of drug affects compliance rates more than the number of drugs. However, not all investigators have found associations with these factors and noncompliance.

Raffoul, Cooper, and Love (1981) have cited data indicating that the most common form of noncompliance to drug regimens in older adults is underuse of prescribed medication. In fact, their own investigation of 67 subjects 60 years or older yielded underuse in 72 percent of the drug misuses uncovered. Similarly, Hemminki and Heikkilä (1975) discovered that, generally, patients have taken prescribed drugs much less frequently than prescribed. Stated reasons for noncompliance most often include no more need for prescribed symptomatic medications and side effects for drugs in which at least one of the pharmacological substances was a proper drug (although this relationship was not statistically significant). They assert that noncompliance to medication protocols may be an active attempt on the part of the consumer to avoid ingesting excessive amounts of drugs.

Cooper et al. (1982) also discovered that in 111 elderly subjects taking prescription medications, 43 percent did not conform to the prescribed regimen. Interestingly, 90 percent of nonadherence was drug underuse and a large proportion of nonadherence (73 percent) was intentional. Additionally, nonadherence was prevalent in those individuals who used two or more pharmacies and two or more physicians.

Of standard doses for older persons, Pfeiffer (1980) has asserted,

> We do not today know what constitutes a standard dosage on any given specific product for an older person, because older persons can respond identically to younger persons in regard to drug dosage, or they may require 75% or 50% or 25% of the usual dosage. That is, virtually every one of any major medications becomes an individual experiment in titration between the physician and his patient. (p. 53).

In light of the evidence pointing to intentional nonadherence on the part of the older person, it is reasonable to assume that they have joined into the spirit of the experiment—often without the benefit of their physician's knowledge and experience.

Rehabilitation Regimens That Don't Consider the Individual.
Weg (1974) has cited data indicating that in comparison to the
18,000 practicing pediatricians in the United States, there were
only 300 geriatricians practicing in 1972. Additionally, Jelly and
Hawkinson (1980) have cited data showing that as recently as
1976, the American Medical Association (AMA) reported no
accredited medical school in the nation that required courses
in geriatrics and only a few that offered electives. A survey tapping
pharmacists' perceptions of major difficulties in geriatric pharmacy yielded as the five most commonly cited problems: inadequate
professional skills or knowledge in geriatrics (29.2 percent of
sample); patient compliance (24 percent); physician functioning,
including drug overprescription (20.2 percent); communication
with elderly (20.2 percent); and lack of professional recognition
(12.9 percent) (Pratt, Simonson, & Lloyd, 1982). Although time
has probably modified some of these situations, they nevertheless
serve as a stark illustration of the level of geriatric health care in
this country.

Central to the lack of geriatric resources is, perhaps, a set of
attitudes about older adults that impede adequate health care.
Butler and Lewis (1982) have labeled these attitudes ageism:
"prejudices and stereotypes that are applied to older persons
sheerly on the basis of their age." Spearheaded by the research
of Tuckman and Lorge (1953), social psychologists and gerontologists have continued to delve into attitudes about older people
held by various facets of society. Older people are almost universally viewed as being unalert, close-minded, nonproductive
members of society, though older adults view themselves as
more adaptive and open-minded than they are given credit for
(Harris & Associates, 1975). Unfortunately, negative views are
held by professionals as well. Spence, Feigenbaum, Fitzgerald,
& Roth (1968) have reported that medical students characterize
older adults as more emotionally ill, disagreeable, inactive, economically burdensome, dependent, dull, socially undesirable,
dissatisfied, socially withdrawn, and disruptive of family harmony
than either adults or youths. Older adults were not seen as anxious
about their futures—perhaps one characteristic that, if observed,
would have evoked some compassion.

Spence et al. (1968) also noted that characterizations of older
adults by medical school seniors did not differ from those of

medical school freshmen. Apparently, the medical school socialization at that time did little to mitigate prevailing stereotypic thinking.

Testimony to the negative stereotyping of older adults abounds in gerontological and recent health care literature (e.g., Shomaker, 1982). Fortunately, these destructive tendencies are beginning to receive broad-scale recognition as evidenced by several recent articles on potential problems in working with a geriatric population and suggestions for improved health care delivery (Gray, 1983; Haynes, Sackett, & Taylor, 1980).

Consequently, prospects for first-rate health care in the future are promising. However, many of these ingrained attitudes have remained stable over the three decades they have been measured, and it will take concerted, dedicated action to dislodge them.

Presently, one can deduce that because of the biases of society at large and of professionals who participate in health care delivery, health services for the elderly suffer. For example, regarding cancer rehabilitation Kennedy (undated) asserts,

> Older patients often have been excluded from chemotherapy clinical trials in order to avoid adverse effects. In most adjuvant chemotherapy studies of Stage II breast cancer, patients over the age of 65 or 70 have been excluded—yet it is in that population that breast cancer is an important disease. The therapeutic effectiveness of chemotherapy in acute nonlymphocytic leukemia emphasizes the importance of including the elderly in clinical studies in order to develop appropriate treatment regimens.

Similarly, Pfeiffer (1974) notes the same tendency in the field of mental health:

> In the field of psychiatry, and in the field of medicine generally, a notion has existed for quite a long time that elderly persons do not respond to treatment. No less a personage that Sigmund Freud stated flatly that elderly patients do not respond to psychotherapy .... He was wrong on this issue ... and his influence has lingered among psychiatrists too long. The plain facts are that the elderly do respond to medical treatment, to drug treatment, and to people treatment, that is psychotherapy, counseling, social interaction and so forth. (p. 34)

The surest way to sabotage the compliance of an older adult is to refrain from giving him or her a chance to follow a prescribed therapeutic regimen. Unfortunately this unwillingness of the health care provider to explore a variety of rehabilitative regimens with older adults is perhaps the most complete form of sabotage. For in the absence of action, the older person cannot even fight back.

Psychological Barriers

Briefly summarized in this section are those psychological barriers that can interfere with the older adult's compliance behavior.

Cognitive Impairment

The prevalence of dementia, including both Alzheimer's type and multi-infarct dementia, is only about five percent of the non-institutionalized population over 65 years of age. Those individuals with senile dementia will exhibit severe learning and memory defects that will seriously interfere with their ability to comply with any therapeutic regimen. For example:

> A woman in her late 70s was referred to an adult day care center by a concerned friend who felt she could no longer meet her ever-increasing needs. The woman was severely organically impaired and was unable to maintain her home or clothe and feed herself without assistance. She had no nearby friends or family, and although her friend was able to shop and provide transportation to physician appointments, she lived too far away to check in on a daily basis. In a routine intake at the center, the staff discovered that the impaired woman had a prescription for hypertension. The friend was encouraged to monitor her drug usage and a few weeks later reported that the woman apparently took the medicine whenever she "found" it. She sometimes "found" her medication several times in a day and sometimes not for days at a stretch.

In this case, the woman's physician was consulted regarding a strategy that would better facilitate compliance to the drug protocol. In the absence of family, close neighbors, or medical personnel at the center who could monitor the medicine, the doctor determined that it would be better to discontinue it than to risk drug misuse. However, this case is extreme in its disposition.

Often, family members, neighbors, or health care personnel can be enlisted to assist organically impaired persons in their medical or rehabilitative procedures and arranging such support is critical when a medical regimen has little flexibility (e.g., insulin-dependent diabetics). Family members are particularly willing to help once they recognize the nature of the disease and begin to learn strategies to manage the impaired person.

Other than the debilitating impact of dementia, older people remain adequately equipped to participate in a rehabilitation regimen. For example, Schaie (1980) has noted that a variety of psychometric measures of intelligence remain stable until 60 years of age, with developmental deficits occurring in older age groups. However, he maintained that the practical significance of these changes may be quite modest. With respect to memory, Storandt (1980) has remarked that older persons do not seem to process new information as deeply as younger persons, and while they do not have problems remembering things once they have learned them, they may have problems learning them well in the first place. Genensky and Zarit (in press) have identified problem areas regarding learning and memory in the older adult. For example, older adults will generally need more time to learn new information. Distractions and information presented at a fast pace can seriously disrupt learning. However, when appropriate compensations are made, memory functioning remains quite adequate (Zarit, 1982).

Depression

Depression is one of the most important psychiatric disorders of late life. In a community-based sample, Blazer and William (1980) have estimated the prevalence of substantial depressive symptomatology to be 14.7 percent. Within this group of depressive older adults, several subgroups emerge. Only 3.7 percent of the depressed group met the criteria for major depressive disorder, several others were judged to be merely dysphoric rather than depressed, and still others (6.5 percent of the depressed sample) had medically related symptoms of depression. For the purposes of this chapter, the high prevalence of depressive symptoms is important because of its behavioral repercussions—feelings dominated by sadness, loss of gratification, constant fatigue, feelings of apathy, behavioral deficits (e.g., psychomotor retardation, diminished social interaction), and somatic complaints (e.g., insomnia) among others. Individuals vary both in terms of symptom pattern and in intensity of specific symptoms. However, the older adult with depressive symptomatology can present quite a serious problem to the health professional who seeks to enlist his or her interest and cooperation with a therapeutic regimen.

Self-Image

The studies on stereotypes of aging discussed above are relevant even within the elderly population. Gerontological literature indicates that older adults often subscribe to the same misconceptions of aging prevalent among the general public. The recent proliferation of media coverage on aging guarantees exposure to stereotypic views of the aging process. Consequently, the current generation of older adults is particularly vulnerable to internalizing these views.

Stereotypic views of aging can be divided into two opposite camps characterized by Shomaker (1982) as the "geriactivist model" and the "incompetence model." The geriactivist model, she suggests, contends that one grows old successfully only to the extent that he or she remains active and involved in the community. Individuals trying to conform to this rigid standard of appropriate aging sometimes believe that they are ill, or generally in poor health, because they cannot always attain this goal. It is not difficult to imagine such an individual seeking help from a physician. Perhaps this situation relates to Pfeiffer's (1980) reports of extreme pressure to prescribe placed by patients on doctors.

The other model of stereotypic thinking—the incompetence model—portrays older adults as a homogeneous group of helpless individuals, according to Shomaker (1982). An extension of this notion is that aging is accompanied by a variety of negative, unavoidable consequences. The extent to which an individual has incorporated this view of aging may be the extent to which his or her compliance is sabotaged by attributing illness to old age and accepting it. An illustration of this point is included in a quote

from Imogen Cunningham (herself an elderly person) in her book
After Ninety (1977):

> She was a famous pianist, and she's ninety-some. She had just under-
> gone an operation for cancer and she had refused further treatment.
> She said, "I might as well die when I'm suppose to," and I said,
> "you're right."

Multiplicity of Problems

The physical, environmental, and psychological barriers noted
above exert a clear influence over individual patients' ability to
comply with specific regimens—especially when the regimen demands that the patient actively engage with health professionals
away from home. Less obvious are the ways in which specific
problems of the older adult (e.g., multiple chronic health problems, reduced financial resources, social isolation) can exacerbate
one another through subtle interplay that not only sabotages
compliance but confuses intervention attempts.

> One 74-year-old patient came to the attention of a low vision clinic
> when her vision impairment became so severe she could no longer ade-
> quately manage her household routine or accomplish errands in the
> community. She was enrolled in a nutrition program for which trans-
> portation was provided. Additionally, the patient received assistance
> from a local hospital concerning her diabetes. An outreach nurse from
> the hospital had even trained the patient's neighbor to fill insulin syringes
> the patient could no longer see. However, she felt apprehensive about
> her future because of her restricted finances and because she felt she
> did not have the skills to survive on her own with her health impair-
> ments. Further, the patient was depressed because of her extreme isola-
> tion. These concerns had a profound affect on her behavior. She often
> missed meals or slept through the appointed hour for her prescribed
> insulin, which exacerbated her already brittle diabetic condition. The
> ensuing illness caused her to miss even more scheduled meals at the
> nutrition site and appointments (e.g., low vision exams and training,
> patient support group to combat isolation, podiatrist appointments) to
> rectify her other problems. Moreover, transportation to these appoint-
> ments was always a problem because she did not always have access to
> someone with a car and found taxis much too expensive to engage on a
> regular basis. The resulting isolation led to more severe depression, a
> greater feeling of hopelessness about her future, and essentially, a repeat
> of the cycle described above.

Clearly, this patient's compliance with both vision and diabetes rehabilitation regimens was precluded by a series of interconnected events that rendered her sickly, apathetic, and functionally homebound. The probability of creating one strategy for combatting all these barriers is low.

In cases such as this, prioritizing patient health care is a critical organizational step. Otherwise, compliance to one rehabilitation program may impede compliance to a more important health need. One strategy used by the low vision clinic in the case above illustrates this point. To combat her isolation and increase her motivation to master her low vision aids, the patient was urged to travel by bus to the clinic for a weekly support group. In the warm weather, bus travel exacerbated her diabetic condition and impeded her compliance to recommendations regarding her primary illness. Furtunately the clinic was able to replace the group support with peer phone calls which in some ways accomplished the same purpose as the support group. This serves to underscore the value of flexible rehabilitation programs that can be modified as other health needs predominate.

ENHANCING COMPLIANCE IN THE OLDER ADULT

This section has two main focuses. First, discussion will center around techniques and strategies the physician or primary health care provider can utilize to enhance compliance. Second, the necessity of mobilizing all resources available to the primary health care provider to maximize the opportunity for compliance in the population of older adults will be explored.

A survey of the health care literature reveals that several suggestions have been offered for making compliance easier from a practical point of view. Some of these suggestions include written instructions (particularly calendars and daily reminder charts) to improve drug compliance (Gabriel, Gagnon, & Bryan, 1977; Wandless & Davie, 1977); reducing waiting time (Haynes et al., 1980); restricting medications to not more than three prescriptions—each having a very distinct color (Fox, 1977); and more generally, keeping programs simple (Haynes et al., 1980).

More complex strategies, such as creating token reinforcement schedules for elderly patients with complex medical regimens, have also proved successful (Dapitch-Miura & Hovell, 1979). However, such protocols often require the participation of a family member or friend—a situation not always possible for the older patient.

Haynes et al. (1980) suggest borrowing from behavior modification principles and linking the rehabilitative regimen (medications, exercise) to an ingrained habit of the individual. For example, if an individual reads the morning newspaper, his or her exercise instructions could be set on top of the newspaper at the breakfast table. Exercising then becomes linked to a daily habit, and the habit becomes a cue for the necessary behavior. Once completed, the necessary behavior is reinforced because the individual can then perform the pleasant task (reading the newspaper).

Along more qualitative lines, the image an older person has of a physician plays an important role in whether or not the older person will seek help. Apparently, technical aspects of medicine or physician performance may be insignificant in encouraging help-seeking behavior. However, the perception of physicians as personally interested in the welfare of patients significantly predicts that an older person will pursue medical help (Nuttbrock & Kosberg, 1980). This notion is important because it underlies the selectivity of older adults relative to their health needs. Moreover, it illustrates the tremendous amount of control older adults exert over the health care services they receive.

Surprisingly, patient participation did not play a major role in the selected survey on compliance. This is unfortunate since the patient constitutes a valuable resource in ensuring compliant behavior (Haynes et al., 1980). Patient participation has been implied in many suggested strategies to improve compliance (e.g., behavioral programs). However, suggestions of an alliance in which the primary health care provider and the patient engage in a frank discussion and mutually agree on a rehabilitation regimen are painfully rare.

Gray (1983) has provided a good framework for a patient-health care provider partnership in his suggestions for improving communication with older adult patients. First, he suggests emphasizing the difference between aging and disease early in the interview, when specific problems are being discussed and when treatment and progress are being evaluated. Additionally, he suggests discussing the possibility of failure with the patient and emphasizing that his or her problems are not necessarily unsolvable even though they might have gotten worse in the past few years. He recommends a positive outlook and setting goals that the older person should be able to attain in order to convince the patient that he or she can succeed. Finally, Gray (1983) suggests that physicians assume a fear of institutionalization on the part of the patient and explicitly state the goal of maintaining the patient at home.

Carried to their logical conclusion (and perhaps beyond their original intent), Gray's (1983) suggestions provide the necessary groundwork for allowing patient-care provider collaboration. First, the patient is educated relative to pertinent disease processes so he or she is less likely to attribute health problems to old age. Second, through skillful interview, the patient identifies facets of the rehabilitative regimen with which he or she may not comply, and alternative plans are created if possible. Finally, the patient and health care provider agree on the same goals (e.g., remaining healthy enough to maintain one's lifestyle in the community), and a partnership is established to attain these goals.

Why is this partnership important? There is some gerontological literature suggesting that while people form impressions of younger persons utilizing a wide variety of distinctive data (e.g., sex, occupation, ethnicity), these distinctive categories are ignored when forming impressions of older adults, and the stereotypes associated with age alone dominate (Bassili & Reil, 1981). This tendency to see older people as a homogeneous group is reflected in much of the research that suggest strategies to enhance compliance without considering differential impact on subgroups of the elderly. Strategies to enhance compliance provide the health professional with powerful tools, but only to the extent that the health care provider matches those tools to patient needs. Allowing older patients to participate in all aspects of health care, from deciding with the health provider an appropriate treatment, to designing a reasonable rehabilitation regimen (again with the health care professional), to deciding what aids and strategies will enhance compliance (e.g., asking a patient how they might fail to comply and posing alternatives) seems a most reasonable and parsimonious route to compliance.

Designing a Program to Enhance Compliance in the Elderly

Even in the best of patient–health care professional relationships, however, problems with compliance may persist. In view of the potential physical, environmental, and psychological barriers previously discussed, it is unrealistic and unreasonable to place the responsibility of ensuring compliance solely on the patient–health professional relationship. Faye and Hood (1975) in discussing compliance to low vision rehabilitation regimens have pursued this line of thought:

> All patients are "motivated"; that is, they want to see, but they may not be able to accept the amount of work it takes to learn to use their vision again in new ways . . . Failure for the low vision person may not be the fault of the patient . . . it may also be the failure of the staff to recognize the patient's basic problem which might be other than physical.

Most gerontologists tend to think along the lines of a multidisciplinary approach to contend with the multitudes of physical and social problems that potentially can affect older adults. Several models of health care delivery are summarized in the gerontological literature (e.g., Brickner et al., 1976; Garetz & Peth, 1974; Giorgi, 1978; Robertson, Griffiths, & Cosin, 1977). The following discussion presents one model of geriatric health care in the form of an outpatient low vision rehabilitation clinic (The Center for the Partially Sighted in Santa Monica, California). From that point of departure, emphasis will be placed on feasible transfers to private practice or to institutions in which a multidisciplinary staff is not possible.

The Center for the Partially Sighted: An Example

The Center for the Partially Sighted is one of the few clinics in the country providing multidisciplinary rehabilitation services for the visually impaired. It was organized in 1978 to aid individuals, the majority of whom are elderly, who have various levels of residual eyesight, the use of which has not been encouraged in other medical settings. The Center's services include evaluation and prescription of visual aids, visual rehabilitation services, and psychological services. It is estimated that nearly two million individuals are partially sighted and many could benefit from the approach of such a center.

Even before a patient reaches the Center, environmental needs are assessed relative to transportation. Most patients are initially escorted to the Center but, occasionally, one of the two staff case coordinators arranges transportation. Upon arriving at the Center, the patient first meets a peer volunteer—someone who has successfully completed the rehabilitation program and who has intimate knowledge of both the problems and potentialities of the new patient. The peer's job is to introduce the new patient to Center services and, implicitly, to serve as a role model to incoming patients. The new patient next sees one of the two staff case coordinators, who will remain the liaison between the patient and the Center. The case coordinator takes a detailed history, including health history, functional limitations resulting from the patient's vision status, and social service needs, and works with the patient to establish rehabilitation goals. (This is particularly important in a low vision setting since aids are often task-specific.)

The case coordinator will then communicate all pertinent information to the low vision specialist and immediately begin to coordinate community resources for any social service needs (e.g., transportation, more activity) the patient may have mentioned. The low vision exam is designed to be comprehensive and takes at least two sessions. To combat financial barriers of older adults, fees are based on a sliding scale and each fee covers a block of time (six months) rather than requiring payment per appointment. This encourages patients to use and reuse the Center until they are satisfied with the rehabilitation outcome.

Following the initial visit with the low vision specialist, a multidisciplinary case conference ensues to plot the rehabilitative course of the patient. By this time, the patient has discussed and negotiated rehabilitation goals with two members of the health care team. Discussion in the case conference focuses primarily on strategies to reduce physical, environmental, and psychlogical barriers to successful rehabilitation. In many ways this translates into ensuring compliance with the low vision regimen.

Resources at hand in a multidisplinary setting are abundant. The case coordinator can provide information and referral services and help patients become reintegrated into active society by providing links with transportation resources, social organizations, and educational/advocacy groups where they can easily find peers. Psychologists are on call to help patients deal with the stress of physical impairment, to clarify their needs relative to the Center, and to help doctor and patient find strategies to make compliance easier. Peer counselors can remain in phone contact with those patients who request such services. Technicians assist patients in learning how to use their aids and in ensuring that the regimen is understood. Finally, case coordinators make frequent follow-up calls to further educate patients, evaluate their progress, and assess their needs.

Center psychologists and optometrists note that these facets of low vision care—working in concert with one another—greatly enhance compliance. In community private practice, however, these resources often appear unobtainable. Because many health providers are not trained to be part of a multidisciplinary team, the organization of multifaceted treatment does not come naturally. Additionally, health and social services in the community are fragmented, and they lack the coordination to make them easily accessible. However, multifaceted treatment is easier to accomplish than it appears.

Of course, each health provider who wants to pursue this approach needs to modify service delivery to meet the needs of his or her practice and patient population. Therefore, specific suggestions would be of limited utility. However, there are some very practical ways to begin.

People from the health provider's own patient population can be utilized as on-site peers and essentially socialize and train new patients to make the most of their health care/rehabilitation. Additionally, peers can make follow-up calls to check on patients' progress. Peer volunteers are a valuable resource and, with proper training, can greatly enhance service delivery.

Even fragmented services can be reached and utilized. The receptionist or other office staff can maintain a file of community services and can even get help in creating that file through existing comprehensive social service organizations. The role of the primary health care provider then becomes one of designating several resources that could best serve the patient. The receptionist would supply the referral. A volunteer, if available, would assist any patient who had difficulty following through on the referral.

SUMMARY

Older adults have a multitude of health problems that make medications and other rehabilitation regimens a part of their everyday lives. For this reason, compliance is a critical element in their health maintenance.

But in addition to their health problems, they face serious physical, environmental, and psychological barriers that impede their ability to comply with health care regimens. The particular impact of these barriers on older adults stands in the way of some otherwise appropriate compliance strategies.

This chapter has explored several practical strategies to enhance compliance in older adults—strategies that consider the special needs and problems of this group. In view of the barriers to compliance in older adults, a multifaceted approach to treatment is recommended when at all possible.

However, the great variability of the older adult population requires the adaptation of these and other strategies to the needs of the individual. Ideally, the cooperation of the older patient should be sought in the design of compliance strategies.

REFERENCES

Atkinson, L., Gibson, I., & Andrews, J. The difficulties of old people taking drugs. *Age, Aging, 6*, 144–150, 1977.

Bassili, J. N., & Reil, J. E. On the dominance of the old-age stereotype. *Journal of Gerontology, 36*(6), 682–688, 1981.

Bierman, E. L., & Brody, H. Our future selves: Report of the panel on biomedical research. (NIH Publication No. 80–1445). *National Advisory Council on Aging*, 1980.

Bild, B. R., & Havighurst, R. J. Senior citizens in great cities: The case of Chicago, Part II. *The Gerontologist, 16*(1), 1976.

Blazer, D., & Williams, C. Epidemiology of dysphoria and depression in an elderly population. *American Journal of Psychiatry, 134*(4), 439–444, 1980.

Brand, F., Smith, R. Medical care and compliance among the elderly after hospitalization. *International Journal of Aging and Human Development, 5*(4), 331–346, 1974.

Brand, F., Smith, R. F., & Brand, P. A. Effect of economic barriers to medical care on patients' noncompliance. *Public Health Reports, 92*(1), 72–78, 1977.

Brickner, P., Janeski, J., Rich, G., Duque, F., Starita, L., LaRocco, R., Flannery, F., & Werlin, S. Home maintenance for the home-bound aged, Part I. *The Gerontologist, 16*(1), 24–29, 1976.

Butler, R. N. Public interest report no. 19—The overuse of tranquilizers in older patients. *International Journal of Aging and Human Development, 7(2)*, 185–187, 1976.

Butler, R. N., & Lewis, M. I. *Aging and mental health: Positive psychosocial approaches* (3rd ed.). St. Louis: C.V. Mosby Company, 1982.

Center for the Partially Sighted, Santa Monica Hospital Medical Center, *Joint progress report to the National Institute of Handicapped Research*, U.S. Department of Education ("Center for the Partially Sighted," #14–P–59166/9) and to the Administration on Aging, U.S. Department of Health and Human Services ("A Comprehensive Community Care System for Partially Sighted Older Persons," #90–A–a600j), June 1980.

Cooper, J., Love, D., & Raffoul, P. Intentional prescription non-adherence noncompliance by the elderly. *Journal of the American Geriatrics Society, 30(5)*, 329–333, 1982.

Cunningham, I. *After ninety*. Seattle: University of Washington Press, 1977.

Curtis, E. Medication errors made by patients. *Nursing Outlook 9*(5), 290–291, 1961.

Dapitch-Miura, E., & Hovell, M. Contingency management of adherence to a complex medical regiment in an elderly heart patient. *Behavior Therapy, 10*, 193–201, 1979.

Decker, T. Survey of hearing loss in older age hospital population. *Gerontologist, 14*, 402–403, 1974.

Faye, E. & Hood, C. (Eds.). *Low vision*. Springfield, IL: Charles C Thomas, 1975.

Federal Council on Aging, U.S. Department of Health and Human Services. *The need for long-term care, information and issues*. (DHHS Publication

(OHDS) 81-20704). U.S. Government Printing Office, Washington, DC, 1981.

Fox, E. M. Drug compliance in the elderly. *British Medical Journal, 1,* 578, 1977.

Gabriel, M., Gagnon, J. P., & Bryan, C. Improved patient compliance through use of a daily drug reminder chart. *American Journal of Public Health, 67*(10), 968–969, 1977.

Garetz, F., & Petn, P. An outreach program of medical care for aged high-rise residents. *The Gerontologist, 14*(5), 404–407, 1974.

Genensky, S. M., & Zarit, S. H. Comprehensive program of low vision services. In A. A. Rosembloom & M. Morgan (Eds.), *Vision and aging: General and clinical perspectives.* Chicago: The Professional Press (in press).

Giorgi, E. Utilizing the health team in the care of the aged. In E. Seymour, (Ed.), *Psychosocial needs of the aged. A health care perspective.* Los Angeles: University of Southern California Press, 1978.

Granick, S., Klehan, M., & Weiss, A. Relationship between hearing loss and cognition in normally hearing aged persons. *Journal of Gerontology, 31*(4), 434–440, 1976.

Gray, M. Communicating with elderly people. In D. Pendleton & J. Hasler, (Eds.), *Doctor-patient communication.* London: Academic Press, 1983.

Harris, L., & Associates. *The myth and reality of aging in America.* Washington, DC: National Council on Aging, 1975.

Hatfield, E. Estimates of blindness in the U.S. *Sight-Saving Review, 43,* 69–80, 1973.

Haynes, R. B., Sackett, D. L., & Taylor, D. W. How to detect and manage low patient compliance in chronic illness. *Geriatrics, 35*(1), 91–97, 1980.

Hemminki, E., & Heikkilä, J. Elderly people's compliance with prescriptions, and quality of medication. *Scandanavian Journal of Social Medicine, 3,* 87–92, 1975.

Hulka, B. S., Cassei, J. C., Kupper, L. L., & Burdette, J. A. Communication, compliance, and concordance between physicians and patients with prescribed medications. *American Journal of Public Health, 66*(9), 847–853, 1976.

Jelly, E., & Hawkinson, W. Geratric eduction in a family practice residency program—an interdisciplinary health-care team approach. *The Gerontologist, 20*(2), 168–172, 1980.

Kennedy, B. J. Cancer and the aging. In *The clinical aspects of aging,* Roche Pharmaceuticals, undated.

Kovar, M. G. Health of the elderly and use of health services. *Public Health Reports, 92*(1), 9–19, 1977.

Lindsay, R. Prescribing for the geriatric patient. In H. B. Haley & P. A. Keenan (Eds.), *Health care of the aging.* Charlottesville, VA: University Press of Virginia, 1981.

Lofholm, P. Self-medication by the elderly. In R. Davis & W. Smith (Eds.), *Health care of the aging.* Charlottesville, VA: University of Virginia Press, 1974.

Lohmann, N. L. Aging and social problems. In H. B. Haley & P. A. Keenan (Eds.), *Health care of the aging,* Charlottesville, VA: University of Virginia Press, 1981.

Lowenthal, M. J. & Robinson, B. Social networks and isolation. In R. H. Binstock & E. Shanas (Eds.), *Handbook of aging and the social sciences.* New York: Van Nostrand Reinhold Company, 1976.

National Center for Health Statistics, *Health in the later years of life: Data from the National Center for Health Statistics.* Washington, DC: U.S. Government Printing Office, 1971.

Neely, E., & Patrick, M. Problems of aged persons taking medications at home. *Nursing Research, 17*(1), 52–55, 1968.

Nuttbroch, L., & Kosberg, J. Images of the physician and help-seeking behavior of the elderly: A multivariate assessment. *Journal of Gerontology, 35(2),* 241–248, 1980.

Ouslander, J. G. Drug therapy in the elderly. *Annals of Internal Medicine, 95(6),* 711–722, 1981.

Pfeiffer, E. Use of drugs which influence behavior in the elderly: Promises, pitfalls, and perspectives. In R. Davis & W. Smith (Eds.), *Drugs and the elderly.* Los Angeles: University of Southern California Press, 1974.

Pfeiffer, E. Pharmacology of aging. In G. Lesnoff-Caravaglia (Ed.), *Health care of the elderly.* New York: Human Sciences Press, 1980.

Pratt, C., Simonson, W., & Lloyd, S. Pharmacists' perceptions of major difficulties in geriatric pharmacy practice. *The Gerontologist, 22*(3), 288–292, 1982.

Raffoul, P. R., Cooper, J. K., & Love, D. W. Drug misuse in older people. *The Gerontologist, 21*(2), 146–150, 1981.

Robertson, D., Griffiths, A., & Cosin, L. A community-based continuing care program for the elderly disabled. *Journal of Gerontology, 32*(3), 334–339, 1977.

Sackett, D., & Snow, J. The magnitude of compliance and noncompliance. In R. B. Haynes, D. Taylor, & D. L. Sackett (Eds.), *Compliance in health care.* Baltimore: Johns Hopkins University Press, 1979.

Schaie, K. W. Cognitive development in aging. In L. Obler & M. Albert (Eds.), *Language and communication in the elderly,* Lexington, MA: Lexington Books, 1980.

Schwartz, D., Wang, M., Zeitz, L., & Goss, M. Medication errors made by elderly chronically ill patients. *American Journal of Public Health, 52(12),* 2018–2029, 1962.

Seidman, H., Silverberg, B. S., & Bodden, A. Probabilities of eventually developing and of dying of cancer. *CA, 28*(1), 33–46, 1978.

Shanas, E., & Maddox, G. L. Aging, health and the organization of health resources. In R. H. Binstock & E. Shanas (Eds.), *Handbook of aging and the social sciences.* New York: Van Nostrand Reinhold Company, 1976.

Shomaker, D. Financial dilemmas. In C. Furukawa & D. Shomaker (Eds.), *Community health services for the aged: Promotion and maintenance.* Maryland: Aspen Publication, 1982.

Spence, D. L., Feigenbaum, E., Fitzgerald, F., & Roth, J. Medical student attitudes toward the geriatric patient. *Journal of the American Geriatric Society, 16,* 976–983, 1968.

Storandt, M. Verbal memory in the elderly. In L. Obler & M. Albert, (Eds.), *Language and communication in the elderly.* Lexington, MA: Lexington Books, 1980.

Tuckman, J., & Lorge, I. Attitudes toward old people. *Journal of Social Psychology, 37,* 249–260, 1953.

Wandless, I., & Davie, J. Can drug compliance in the elderly be improved? *British Medical Journal, 1,* 578, 1977.

Weg, R. Drug interaction with the changing physiology of the aged: Practice and potential. In R. Davis & W. Smith (Eds.), *Drugs and the elderly.* Los Angeles: University of Southern California Press, 1974.

Zarit, S. H. Affective correlates of self-reports about memory of older people. *International Journal of Behavioral Geriatrics, 1,* 25–34, 1982.

8

The Eye of the Beholder: Staff Perceptions of Noncompliance

Alexis M. Nehemkis

How often do we consider whether our biases and our concerns of the moment—and even our motives for becoming physicians, nurses, or psychologists—are affecting the people we treat? It is important to ask ourselves whether we are identifying true problem areas for the patient or are overemphasizing an area because of our own life situation. Is our judgment of a patient's cooperativeness based on objective behavioral indices or does it reflect our own needs for how patients *should* behave?

Staff expectations of patients are at least partially a function of how we perceive or evaluate the life changes and losses that occur in the patients with whose care we are charged. We ask ourselves in trying to determine how patients behave, what does being on dialysis or undergoing chemotherapy do to the patient? What does he or she go through? What are important as opposed to unimportant changes for this patient? The answers to these questions will strongly affect the themes we emphasize in treating these patients and the areas we examine most closely in anticipating problems.

What I propose to do in this chapter is to draw together some of the thematic threads from various areas which point to the way in which bias can color a hospital staff's expectations and required standards for patient behavior. Staff attitudes and expectancies do influence the behavior of patients on a treatment unit. Staff bias is explored from the perspective of bias operating in the judgment process, resulting in one patient being labeled as compliant and another as noncompliant. Staff bias as the wrong criterion measure of compliance is also discussed.

Some of the cases and areas I draw upon, by the very nature of this topic, must remain suggestive: with certain patient groups (e.g., hemodialysis) we can demonstrate a direct link between these expectations and patient compliance. With other groups (e.g., oncology, surgical patients) whose manifest compliance rates are high, the link is indirect, and patient compliance in this context refers to the degree to which patients conform to unwritten norms of adaptive sick-role behavior which staff comes to expect.

Unless otherwise indicated, the term staff as used in this chapter refers to all of the component personnel of a ward system: the housestaff (interns and residents), fellows, the attendings, allied medical disciplines (social workers, dieticians, consulting psychologists, physical therapists), but especially, the RNs and their assistants. Because of the nurses' more constant exposure to the problems on a ward (they are present for an eight-hour shift in contrast to the physicians' sporadic presence—sometimes only a matter of minutes), our observations reflect this awareness.

STAFF VERSUS PATIENT PERCEPTIONS OF LIFE CHANGES EXPERIENCED WITH CHRONIC ILLNESS

The burden of the day-in and day-out care in a chronic care setting falls heavily on the nursing staff. In addition, nurses who deal with the chronic care patient tend to be given more direct responsibilities in overseeing the management of the patients. As a result, nurses may find themselves faced with the dilemma of having to negotiate their way between physicians' rigid prescriptions for care and their own appreciation of the nuances of some patients' failure to comply. The reasons for staff expectations and attitudes discussed in this chapter may be traced, in part, to their predicament.

Previous research has identified significant discrepancies between the ways in which chronically ill patients and their medical caretakers tend to perceive life changes associated with the illness

(Blank, 1979; Gerber, 1980; Hanson & Franklin, 1976; Nehemkis, et al., 1984). Hanson & Franklin (1976), for example, found staff to be mistaken in assuming that sex is frequently the most devastating of all functional losses to spinal cord injured males.

Staff members in a rehabilitation service were asked to rank the importance of functional losses as they believed their quadriplegic patients would. The areas included normal use of legs, normal control of bowel and bladder function, normal feeling in use of sexual organs, and normal use of arms and hands. The patients were asked to rank the same items. The majority of these spinal cord injury patients ranked sex as being the least important of the major functional losses. Staff members, on the other hand, viewed the loss of sexual function as substantially more important to the patients than the patients did themselves. Staff were found to undervalue, as compared to patients, the relative value of the functional loss of their limbs.

A similar study was conducted by Gerber (1980) that compared the perceptions of dialysis nurses and patients undergoing dialysis treatment with respect to nine areas of life changes or loss often cited in the clinical literature as significant for patients on renal dialysis (e.g., dietary alterations, increased financial burdens, decreased sexual activity). Staff tended to overemphasize the relative importance of changes in family relationships and sexual functioning while underestimating patients' sense of loss due to dietary restrictions, travel limitations, and inability to complete routine household chores. Gerber did not conclude that sex and family issues were unimportant to these patients but rather that other aspects of their changed lifestyle were perceived by the patients as more important. For the patient who must live with the myriad stresses and difficulties associated with being on dialysis, it is, perhaps, the most simple, daily activities— the ones usually taken for granted—that are of most significance. Such changes have been observed by Yalom (1980) in his work with cancer patients. His patients consistently reported shifts in life priorities which were evidenced by a living in the present, fewer interpersonal concerns, a deeper appreciation of the elemental facts of life—overall, an inner directed shift (Yalom, 1980).

For those suffering from disabilities, it is not uncommon for the world to shrink and for areas of meaning and significance to narrow and turn inward. The reassessment of life priorities when faced with a chronic or terminal illness apparently stems—although it is not necessarily well articulated by patients—from an unavoidable confrontation with their mortality. This rearrangement of life emphasis is difficult for the healthy individual (i.e., professional staff) to comprehend. These findings served to reinforce the salience of subjective, internal changes and losses that coincide with the onset of severe chronic disability—losses often taken for granted by the healthy.

Alice Stewart Trillin (1981) has expressed similar ideas most eloquently in her discourse to doctors on being a cancer patient. A year after she had a cancerous lung removed, doctors asked her what she was most concerned about. Her reply was "garden peas":

> Not the peas themselves, of course, though they were particularly good that year. What was extraordinary to me after that year was that I could again think that peas were important, that I could concentrate on the details of when to plant them and how much mulch they would need instead of thinking about platelets and white cells. I cherished the privilege of thinking about trivia. Thinking about death can make the details of our lives seem unimportant, and so, paradoxically, they become a burden . . . . (p. 701).

This phenomenon of heightened preoccupation with apparent trivia has been observed in one other (nonillness) situation of great stress and turmoil—war. A pilot of the Royal Air Force serving with a night-flying fighter squadron in 1939 observed the following in a letter to his brother written from the fighting front:

> A protective mechanism develops which enables one to concentrate on unimportant events. For example, the high spot of our day at camp is the arrival of cake for tea. It comes every day from Lyons, and the question is whether it will be a nauseous pink, a dirty white, or a camouflage brown. This having been ascertained, we sink back in to a comatose condition to await what the next day will bring. (Straight, 1983, p. 145)

These value changes which occur during the period of an adjustment to a stressful condition—such as a chronic illness—make difficult the communication between insider (i.e. patient) and outsider (i.e. staff). Staff judgments of how patients should behave become confounded by significant, yet often unspoken, differences in life priorities. For the healthy individual, a future orientation is common, but for the individual with a shortened and functionally limited life span, new priorities develop—priorities often viewed as unimportant by the healthy outsider.

A recent study by Blank (1979) illustrates value changes such as those described above which may occur with cancer patients. The author examined the replies of nurses and advanced cancer patients about the perceived need of the patients. Results of the study confirmed that nurses tend to overemphasize certain patient needs as being more important than do the patients. Thus, the needs perceived by the patient may be ignored.

To better delineate these differences between staff and patients in the perception of patient needs, we asked 26 cancer patients, five oncologists, and 10 nursing staff to rank in order of personal importance to the patients 14 areas of life changes or loss commonly alluded to in the psychosocial oncology literature (Nehemkis, Gerber, & Charter, 1984). Our findings indicated that physicians consistently identify certain losses as very important to their patients (e.g. self-care activities, lessened energy level), while the patients did not view these losses as especially important. In this respect, these physicians are different than the dialysis staff who consistently underestimated the patient's sense of loss owing to an altered mobility, self-care, and daily routine. Similarly, the nursing staff consistently predicted certain losses to be important. Unlike their counterparts on the dialysis unit, the oncology nursing staff predicted that changes in physical appearance would be more devastating than did the patients.

Interestingly, patients with advanced cancer did not single out any one item or cluster of items as having overriding importance in their lives. It appears that the importance of any particular loss or life change is very much a matter of individual differences. Unlike the patients with end-stage renal disease or spinal cord injury, no immutable themes characterize the perceptions of advanced cancer patients as a group. In sum, cancer patients do not identify any single loss or life change as of major consequence, whereas the staff assumes they will.

The thematic hierarchy of life changes and losses, so evident in the dialysis and spinal cord injury patients, did not emerge in this patient population. One explanation for the striking lack of variability in the patients' average responses may lie in the characteristics of the disease: Cancer, unlike end-stage renal disease or traumatic myelopathy, is not one disease, but many, characterized by a variable course and variable prognosis. The significant individual variability of both the course and prognosis of cancer may also sensitize the staff to refrain from extremes in stereotyping patient concerns, as has been found with more homogeneous groups of dialysis or spinal cord injury patients. Nonetheless, certain staff biases do evolve even in relation to this diverse patient group.

THE IMPORTANCE OF PAIN IS OVERRATED

While the clinical literature on cancer persists in assigning particular salience to pain in the process of coping with the disease, our results do not confirm this conclusion. The significance of pain must pale in the face of more profound psychological and existential issues invoked by the cancer predicament—the meaning of the life one has lived, the imminent loss of everyone and everything ever held dear, and the anticipation of one's own death. As expected, staff members overrated the importance of pain in the experience of the advanced cancer patient.

Staff biases and misperceptions can result in selective attention to certain complaints, thereby lending them a legitimacy not accorded others. The operation of subtle bias permits the staff to accept a patient's complaints of pain at face value and, perhaps, to imbue them unwittingly with a larger significance than that with which they are offered. Eager for the opportunity to ventilate their feelings and not wishing to disappoint their caretakers, patients are prone to contribute the existence of pain to conform with their view of the staff's expectations.

Overemphasis on certain issues, such as pain, may reflect the tendency of the staff to translate a patient's emotional and psychological distress into physical symptoms more readily treatable by the conventional medical and nursing technology. Indeed our experience as consultants to cancer unit staff has revealed that such a process of overemphasizing physical components of the patient's predicament takes place. Although such a process is understandable in view of the training and professional role of the medical staff, the implications for the patient are that certain fundamental emotional concerns may be selectively ignored in favor of such concrete problems. As noted in an earlier article (Wright & Nehemkis, 1983), intervention designed to relieve organic symptoms—pain, for instance—may prove futile if such symptoms do not represent the patient's true dilemma. Compartmentalization in treatment of cancer patients and an overemphasis on symptom management may serve to enhance the credibility of the physician/nurse's acute care role at the expense of the true concerns of the patient.

In a poignant commentary by a physician with end-stage renal disease who has been, in his words, both "a voyeur and a partaker in human suffering," Calland (1972) outlined a similar process of overemphasis on the physical components of the patient's predicament by the nephrologist who cares for the patient on dialysis:

> Patients on dialysis are accustomed to being told by the doctor, "You are doing fine"—usually after the latest measurement of electrolytes and creatinine. The patient then thinks to himself, "If I'm doing fine, why do I feel so rotten?" . . . . Eventually, the time comes when the patient complains of nothing, and the doctor is thus wholly unaware of these symptoms, just as he is unaware of the other (marital, financial, and social) difficulties that the patient is experiencing . . . . The doctor is thus at a terrible disadvantage of his own making—the terrible disadvantage of having knowledge of his patients' feelings about illness and treatment concealed from him. (p. 335)

It is evident from each of these examples of the differing views of life changes and loss as perceived by patients and staff that if priority were assigned those areas which the professional staff believed were of most importance to their patients, the issues the patients considered most relevant would be overlooked. The results of the four studies presented in this section imply that a biased staff (1) may compromise the patient emotionally or otherwise deny the patient total care, through selective wrong therapeutic emphasis; and (2) may deleteriously affect the ambience on the unit. It would seem relatively uncontroversial to assert that spinal cord injured patients, end-stage renal disease patients, and cancer patients in the advanced stage of the disease should be evaluated on an individual basis by a staff as unencumbered as possible by its own priorities and preconceptions. For staff–patient communication to be therapeutic, it is essential that there exist a certain degree of shared perspective between healer and healed.

EXAMPLES FROM AN ONCOLOGY UNIT

Concentrating one kind of patient with serious illness and a high mortality rate on one ward can provoke a major emotional stress in the staff: they have fewer patients with recoverable illness with which to counterbalance the emotional strain occasioned by the terminally ill patient. Time does not permit for sufficient ventilation of staff feelings nor is there group permission for such open expression of emotion on an oncology unit, with its frequent rotation of housestaff, heavy concentration of seriously ill patients, considerable patient turnover, and high death rate. Scapegoating (as well as numerous lesser, short-lived instances, involving projection of staff feelings, misperceptions, misplaced concern, and selective inattention) under such conditions is an expedient mechanism for release of tensions and enhancing group (staff) cohesion. In previous articles on this mechanism and variants of the scapegoating process (Nehemkis, Stampp, & Amaral, 1981-1982; Yeargan & Nehemkis, 1982), we noted that when the staff felt threatened in some way, it would cast about for a target, creating and maintaining distorted perceptions in an effort to reduce ward tension. From our vantage point as observers of this system over the course of several years, although the target has changed and the process varied, the underlying mechanism, nevertheless, persists. Individuals singled out for hostile projections have been drawn from among the ward staff's own ranks, or from the patients. Previous observations on the system characteristics of the cancer ward contain a discussion of the dialectical features reflected in distorted staff judgments about three areas in particular:

1. Perceived overinvolvement or underinvolvement of family members in a patient's care: Staff members will complain of underinvolvement—"They're not there enough!" We, in turn, receive referrals oscillating between both ends of this spectrum. It seems as if in the general perception of the staff few families fall into the appropriate area of involvement.

2. The mood spectrum: Staff judgments about the mood spectrum also reflect dialectical features. Patients are seen as either too depressed or too happy—as if there were a delicate, albeit rarely achieved, balance that patients were supposed to have along this spectrum.

In his comment on the chapters on "Coping with Cancer" in Cullen et al. (1976), Pearson offers a similar admonishment:

> We are so used to thinking that a patient who is depressed, sad or crying is not entitled to be that way, and that we must modify that mood somewhat, usually so that we, or the nursing staff, will feel more comfortable . . . . I think we as professionals find it difficult to allow a normal period for anticipatory grief, for mourning for the lost function or part, and for extending the limits of what we might consider normal and appropriate depression. (p. 284)

3. Denial and acceptance: A similar dialectic appears to be operating along the denial—acceptance dimension. We receive a number of referrals for denial. Most of these reflect the staff's mistaken tendency to confuse behavior or communication which represent pathological denial of reality with those which reflect a patient's selective inattention and way of coping which may have positive adaptational value. Interestingly, however, we also receive an occasional referral when a patient appears to have achieved

that rarer stage of acceptance. The patient has accepted his impending death, but the staff recasts this act of serenity and misinterprets it as giving up.

The identified problem patient or relative becomes a screen for the projection of staff feelings along the dialectical dimensions just outlined. In such situations there may be scapegoating of the patient or family member by the staff who provides a highly distorted version of the situation.

Another, though mirror-image, variation of the scapegoating process occurs when, from time to time, the staff rallies around a patient who, it would appear, evokes within them a disproportionately empathic response. The staff as a whole becomes deeply invested in this patient who becomes for them a "project" which serves to divert their focus away from the constant presence of death. Thus, staff bias is not invariably objectionable—it may sometimes work to the patient's advantage.

NONCOMPLIANCE RESULTING FROM INCONGRUENT EXPECTATIONS

The following case, though not involving a matter of life and death or institutionalized debilitating illness, nevertheless illustrates the destructive sequence which can follow when patient and health professional have very disparate perceptions of the chief complaint. In this case the incongruity between the expectation of the patient and the staff member's definition of the problem virtually ensures that noncompliance will be the result.

A 70-year-old widow who had retired with her husband to California came to a low vision center because of increasingly poor vision. She was seen by an optometrist who evaluated her problem as advanced macular degeneration, which results in loss of central vision, and prescribed an elaborate set of low vision aids (including a high-power magnification reading lens and microscopic spectacles). The objective was to restore reading to its assumed deserved place of importance in the patient's life. She was given the usual instruction that accompanies prescription of these devices, and the devices themselves were enthusiastically presented to her. At the time of her next scheduled follow-up appointment, it was, therefore, a surprise to the optometrist when the patient seemed totally disheartened and had evidently given up any attempt at practic-

ing with the vision aids. At this point, such a patient might be lost to
follow up and written off as a treatment failure due to noncompliance.

The optometrist was operating under the assumption that it
is vital for people to read and that this patient wanted to resume
reading books. In fact, the patient was not an avid reader and had
no compelling interest in reading and, hence, books were of minor
interest. Indeed, her objective, at this stage of life—though she had
been unable to articulate it with sufficient clarity and force to
alter the optometrist's assumptions about what was important
to her—was to be able to read newspaper headlines, perhaps a
short news story, a shopping list, and item prices in the super-
market. What she actually received was a set of sophisticated
devices (intended for the avid reader of books) which can be
unwieldy and difficult to master unless the recipient exerts a
great deal of perseverance and the kind of commitment of time
and patience that only someone with a passionate devotion to
books would put forth. The devices required to meet her objectives (to scan newspaper headlines and read grocery lists) are less
sophisticated (e.g., a small pocket magnifier which can be worn
around the neck) and thus more easily mastered than the devices
with which she was provided.

Compliance was fatally sabotaged from the outset because of
the discrepancy between her objectives and the expectations of
the optometrist. In short, the optometrist prescribed devices
with his own intellectual needs in mind rather than those of his
patient. Closer attention must be given to the staff–patient relationship, the nature of the expectations each has, and the congruence and mutuality of such expectations. There must be congruence between the doctor's approach to therapy and the patient's attitudes toward the problem and expectations from
treatment. When that congruence is lacking, noncompliance is
the ineluctable result.

PATIENT COMPLIANCE AS A FUNCTION OF STAFF ATTITUDES AND EXPECTATIONS

Numerous studies across a spectrum of research areas combine
to indicate unequivocally that individuals are responsive to what
is overtly or covertly expected to them. Therapist prognostic

expectancies influence patient progress (Goldstein & Shipman, 1961). The unplanned influence of the experimenter's expectancies on research subjects is well known and the basis for at minimum double-blind designs (Rosenthal, 1963). Much the same phenomenon has been demonstrated by Masling (1964) in the psychological testing context; by Orne (1959) in his studies of demand characteristics associated with the induction of hypnosis; by Hyman, Cobb, Feldman, Hart, and Stember (1954) in their studies of interview bias effects in survey research. It is widely accepted that in treating hospitalized patients, relationships with the ward staff are important; moreover, the attitudes and messages of nursing staff, who spend much more time with patients than do physicians, are critical in influencing patients' expectations and acceptance of treatment (Gillmore & Hill, 1981).

A direct link between staff attitudes and expectations and patient behavior and compliance has been demonstrated in hemodialysis patients by the work of De-Nour (1981). Patients' adjustment and compliance with the diet is hindered by two types of antitherapeutic attitudes on the part of the medical staff: lack of staff agreement about the desired or expected behavior and unrealistically high staff expectations for patient adjustment, which even "good" patients cannot fulfill.

Recalling the earlier discussion of cancer patients, unrealistic expectations come into play along the mood spectrum or when staff mistakenly feels a patient is denying or giving up. A certain level of depression is apparently understood by this ward staff to be normal. Disagreement among the nursing staff arises most often, we later learned, over whether patients were sufficiently depressed to warrant consultation. Patient compliance in this context refers to the degree to which patients conform to "unwritten norms" of adaptive behavior which staff expects. This underscores the importance of establishing appropriate reliable criteria for satisfactory adjustment, adaptation—in a word, compliance.

WHAT DETERMINES A STAFF'S VIEW OF COMPLIANCE?

It would seem that the crucial determinant of staff's judging a dialysis patient, for instance, to be noncompliant is probably not a simple, linear weighting and totaling of separate mental notations regarding the patient's own care of the blood access, observance of appointments, taking of medicine, reporting of changes in physical condition, limiting of physical activity as directed by staff, observance of the prescribed diet, and so forth. Instead it probably draws upon something of a profoundly personal nature, not even fully articulated by the clinician himself.

There is much suggestive evidence that this is the case. In one of the early studies of bias in the assessment of patients on chronic dialysis, De-Nour and Czaczkes (1974) found that "some of the nephrologists assess how well a patient is doing mostly by his compliance to the diet, functioning at work and emotional condition. *Other nephrologists give greater importance to other* (even more subjective) *facets of the patient's condition"* emphasis added) (p. 217). Moreover, as De-Nour (1981) has observed more recently, "just to be well adjusted was not sufficient to gain the (dialysis) staff's acceptance. Patients' actual behavior in the unit—good behavior, cooperation, and being interesting to talk to—were important factors in acceptance, while seeking attention and being troublesome led to rejection" (p. 127).

Relevant also is Lorber's (1975) research on the reaction of medical personnel to hospitalized patients. Patients who were stoical, uncomplaining, cooperative, and did not interrupt the unit's work flow were categorized as "good patients." "Problem patients" were those who were uncooperative, who complained a good deal, were anxious and overemotional. Good patients were less likely to receive time and attention from the staff; they were also more likely to be discharged with dispatch. (The full extent of the psychological liabilities of good patient behavior is well delineated in an article by Taylor, 1979.) Patients admitted for cancer surgery were the most likely to be categorized by housestaff and nurses as good patients. The relevance of Lorber's work resides in the implied equation of "good" with compliant and "problem" with noncompliant. The significance of this study lies in the implications of staff labeling certain patients as good. These individuals are subsequently denied access to potential sources of professional support and time and attention early in the diagnostic treatment sequence. Good (cancer) patients' psychosocial needs go unrecognized and unattended. The significance of this failure of recognition is that lack of a support system, including doctors who are seen as less helpful and concerned, is a risk factor for emotional vulnerability and distress at a later stage of the illness (e.g., Weisman, 1979).

Gerber, Falke, and Ralidis (1984) examined a variety of factors that staff use to judge a patient's compliance. A global rating of compliance on 33 patients was made by each R.N. in a renal dialysis unit. Nurses rated the patients on social-psychological dimensions such as likeability, perceived similarity to the individual nurse, friendliness, independence, dependence etc. Nurses' job attitudes were also assessed. Objective biochemical indicators of compliance were gathered from the medical chart. Results showed that more compliant patients were perceived as more likeable and more similar to staff than noncompliant patients. Staff labeling of a patient as compliant or noncompliant was not related to commonly accepted objective, biochemical criteria for compliance. Social-psychological factors accounted for more of the variance in predicting whether a patient was labeled as compliant than did biochemical evidence.

STAFF EXPECTATIONS FOR INDEPENDENCE: COVERT DEMANDS FOR DEPENDENCY

In a fascinating article on the structure and pattern of staff–patient relationships in the dialysis setting, Alexander (1976) illustrates the progression of a double bind. Independent behavior is both demanded and denied. The staff directive to be independent subsumes all lesser directives regarding dietary and fluid intake, all rules of self-care, including hygiene and asepsis, regular and punctual attendance for treatment, and the like. Paradoxically, "be independent" is negated by the caretakers and by the hemodialysis treatment context. Institutionalized medical caretaking retains for itself responsibility for decisions related to the care and treatment of patients. Information that would permit independent decision making by patients is usually screened and restricted. (See also Spradlin & Porterfield, 1980.)

A case in point was the finding that eight of the nine black patients in our study (Gerber, Nehemkis, Farberow, & Williams, 1981) were rated into the uncooperative group. The black patients on dialysis felt less valued and less appreciated by their families and friends. As a result they depended more on the hospital, its staff, and their fellow patients. Their dependency was viewed negatively by the medical and nursing staff who had the treatment goal of making the patients as self-sufficient and as independent of the hospital as possible. (This led, of course, to their being rated less cooperative.)

Such personality factors and structurally inherent double binds are not peculiar to the dialysis setting and may operate to cause abuse and noncompliance in any chronic medical setting or treatment unit. Observations of the spinal cord injured patient suggest that his self-destructive behavior appears to give him some sense of power and control, which helps him to overcome feelings of inadequacy and helplessness. The same theme of staff expectations for independence while demanding dependency applies to this population and is embodied in a variant of Alexander's "be independent" directive—"be normal." Productivity, family cohesion, emotional stability, the reattainment of pre-illness lifestyle are examples of staff expectations for spinal cord injury patients. The secondary injunction is of the sort "you are not normal," and staff are caught in the dilemma, on the one hand, of endorsing the rehabilitation ideal and, on the other, harboring misgivings that it may not be fair to demand this ideal from a patient whose functional autonomy is greatly impoverished and of whom they demand simultaneously rigorous health maintenance within a slim margin (Nehemkis & Groot, 1980).

DESIGNING AN INTERVENTION PROGRAM TO COUNTER STAFF BIAS ON THE SPECIALTY CARE UNIT

The search for stable characteristics of the patient that will deepen our understanding of compliance phenomena or enable us to better predict noncompliance has failed. While the evidence suggests that the dynamics of compliance are configural and ever-changing, staff are unaccustomed to think of anything other than static patient characteristics as reasons for noncompliance (e.g., Davidson, 1976; DiMatteo & DiNicola, 1982; Stimson, 1974). This contains shades of Kasl's (1975) paradox: compliance—traditionally investigated from the physician's, not the patient's perspective, with the patient, not the physician, the one invariably studied.

The Hemodialysis Unit: An Example

From the earliest days of our involvement with the dialysis unit at the Long Beach VA Medical Center, it was apparent that consultation to the nursing staff, which is charged with the day-to-day running of the unit, would be a critical task. Much time was spent monitoring the nursing staff's activities and attempting to enhance their effectiveness in dealings with patients. One of the first interventions involved establishing a weekly group meeting with all of the dialysis nurses. A prime interest was to mesh the orientation of this group with the personality styles of the nurses with whom we were to work to ensure a greater usefulness to this staff than the feeling-oriented, cathartic group paradigm frequently espoused in the consultation-liaison literature (Czaczkes & De-Nour, 1978; Rogers, 1975). These nurses typically coped with the stresses of their work by employing defenses which made them appear more intellectually detached, rational, and controlled. While not manifesting coldness toward their patients, these nurses had developed, perhaps through exposure, a detached concern, limiting the extent of their emotional involvement with patients and families.

In the weekly meetings with the nursing staff, we have always stressed the psychological and social situational context for behavior in an effort to enhance empathy and a more sophisticated appreciation of the plight and predicament of difficult patients in particular. By encouraging the group members to search the environment, as it were, for explanations of noncompliant behaviors, we hoped to counteract their tendency to commit the fundamental attribution error (Ross, 1977)—to ascribe noncompliance to personality defects on the part of the patient. Despite staff receptivity to our consultation strategy, the view of noncompliance as something lodged within the patient is not easily routed. Our efforts have been directed at discouraging this tendency to overattribute all manifestations of noncompliance to immutable personality traits, while refocusing the staff's attention on conceptually more meaningful and more easily changed sources in the social or interpersonal environment.

The danger, of course, of excessive internal trait attributions is that they (1) serve to absolve staff members of responsibility for examining their interaction with patients as potential stimuli for noncompliant actions, and (2) eventually generate a self-fulfilling prophecy.

Liaison consultants may be able to enhance the effectiveness of such interventions by applying standardized information gathering procedures and by adapting systematic feedback and change strategies that have proven successful in other settings. And, of course, nurses should be allowed a regular time to explore pertinent issues that affect their care of patients.

A COGNITIVE-BEHAVIORAL APPROACH TO RESTRUCTURING STAFF ATTITUDES AND EXPECTATIONS

We are experimenting with the application to our staff group of a sequence of procedures adapted from Turk, Meichenbaum, and Genest's (1983) cognitive-behavioral approach to pain management. Staff members record their perceptions of different problem patients' noncompliant actions, to sensitize them to cues that may be associated with the behavior. In addition, they may also record their own thoughts and feelings evoked by the patients' actions. These observations are then used to generate staff discussions of the potential impact of their reactions to the patient on that patient's behavior and interpersonal factors that can serve to maintain the noncompliance. Throughout the initial phase of data gathering and assessment, a conceptual model for compliance is gradually introduced, reviewed, and reiterated with the aim of encouraging staff to adopt a way of looking at noncompliance that inherently allows for change. The consultants work with the nursing staff to develop a more differentiated view of the problem and systematically reconceptualize their attitudes, perceptions, and attributions of noncompliant behavior. Particular attention is paid to each nurse's cognitions about patient non-compliance. Their cognitions may then be incorporated into specific interventions, the consultants modifying those which are irretrievably antitherapeutic and capitalizing on or reframing those which may be useful.

THE TEAM TREATMENT CONCEPT: A CAUTIONARY NOTE

In the preceding pages we sketched our ideas about how a cognitive-behavioral approach might be adapted for group use with nursing staff on a medical treatment unit, to deal more effectively with staff resistance and attempt a systematic cognitive restructuring of their views of patient behavior, including noncompliance. Our enthusiasm for the possibilities of adapting and tailoring this approach to enhance the effectiveness of staff as a group is tempered, however, by some basic reservations about the efficacy and wisdom of patient management by group. We know that group decisions tend to be more extreme or more risky than individual decisions made in isolation. Something occurs in the process of interpersonal confrontation and the give-and-take of a group discussion that generates a decision to favor more risky alternatives. The clinical implications of these findings (e.g., Stoner, 1961; Wallach, Kogan, & Bem, 1964; Wallach & Kogan, 1965) are somewhat disquieting in the context of the myriad decisions about patient care generated by team treatment—an approach which has been fashionable for some-time. As the work of these social psychologists has demonstrated, conditions are present in the team meeting that foster a diffusion of responsibility and generate a shift toward more extreme or risky decisions that can become the breeding ground for destructive staff bias and, in turn, have drastic effects upon what treatment is recommended and what patient options are disallowed.

Consider the case of a 61-year-old married veteran who had been a patient on in-center dialysis for several years. He was well liked by the nurses who had often gone out of their way to accommodate him in little extra ways. Because of his nonservice connected status, his eligibility for in-center dialysis was being reclassified, and so when the continuous ambulatory peritoneal dialysis (CAPD) program was established at the medical center, he expressed an interest. He and his wife investigated it thoroughly and made a good case for his suitability for transfer into this program. It was, therefore, a surprise to us when the patient's announced desire to remain on hospital-based dialysis at this medical center evoked real dismay in the dialysis staff. Apparently his inquiries about CAPD had been blocked by the bureaucratic rules of the program which he did not technically meet. The patient had a tracheostomy, which was well cared for, but which is a risk factor for peritonitis—a worrisome complication of this method of dialysis. The program also requires that patients be able to open the bag which he could not do unaided. Staff did not take into account that his wife, who did not work outside the home, was available and willing to assist him with these manipulations. Staff would not alter its criteria. His enthusiasm first for the new program and then his express desired to remain a patient at the center evoked real consternation in the staff. One afternoon, one of the nurses happened to see him in the offices of a veteran's organization inquiring about his legal rights of access to the CAPD program. The depth of the staff's feeling was reflected in this R.N.'s subsequent report to the others: "We've got to stand by our decision!" Once he had appeared to question their authority, battle lines were drawn, with staff intransigent and unwilling to consider some options that were truly available to this couple.

While subjective staff conceptions of the patient's problem just as often work in a positive direction, in this example the staff response fostered an "us versus them" attitude leading to decisions perhaps not in the best interest of the patient. The unique circumstances of the patient's life were ignored in favor of maintaining rules and setting limits. Such situations inevitably lead to ever-escalating patient–staff antagonism.

CONCLUSION: IS PERFECT COMPLIANCE A NECESSARY AND SUFFICIENT CONDITION FOR ADJUSTMENT TO CHRONIC ILLNESS?

Elsewhere it was observed that the more cooperative dialysis patients were invested in the hospital staff, rather than in fellow patients, for feelings of worth. In other words they apparently derived a significant sense of their self-esteem and self-worth from their relationships with doctors and nurses on the unit. At that time it was suggested that this might represent a greater degree of identification with the positive aspects of the medical regimen (represented by staff) rather than with the negative aspects of the illness (represented by other patients). The design of that study does not permit a definitive interpretation, but upon further reflection, it seems equally plausible that the more compliant patients who were emotionally invested in their caretakers were the patient equivalent of "teacher's pet"—their compliance was motivated by the desire to please. As Tagliacozzo and Mauksch (1972) have observed, pleasing the doctor and nurse by behaving properly—doing what one is told and not making trouble—becomes for the hospitalized patient a chief role obligation.

This leads us to question whether such exemplary compliance to please the staff, perhaps, is the most effective way to deal with chronic illness and disability. In posing this question, we reiterate a theme suggested in Chapter 5—that, paradoxically, faultless compliance may not always be in the service of optimal adjustment to chronic illness. To what extent is compliance the healthiest approach? Is it better for a patient occasionally to question the treatment, to be, in essence, a thoughtful participant with his physician, than to follow a prescribed regimen blindly? Taylor (1979) has advanced a compelling argument that the good patient role may be not only undesirable from the patient's perspective, but that because of a whole host of behavioral, cognitive, affective, and physiological concomitants of this pattern, good patients may run actual health risks at the hands of the staff who care for them and so label them.

It will be recalled that in the preceding discussion we urged the establishment of appropriate, reliable criteria for adjustment— the operative word here being appropriate—which in the case of chronic disease or disability must be a dynamic process. White's (1974) notion of successful adaptation as "a striving towards acceptable compromise" more nearly suggests a judicious testing of the limits than blind, unquestioning adherence.

The relationship between degree of compliance to the medically defined norms of treatment and overall adjustment to the illness may be a curvilinear one. In this view, it is not the absolute degree of compliance that is the most important determinant of an optimal and satisfying adjustment. On one end of a continuum would fall those patients whose infractions of the regimen are severe and patently self-destructive. On the other end are the "model patients" who are perfectly compliant, or nearly so. Those who are in the middle of this continuum and who exhibit occasional, minor trial-and-error, perhaps, self-correcting non-compliant deviations from the prescribed regimen are most well adjusted. Clearly, it remains for future studies to provide a firm empirical base for the association between compliance and adjustment to disability.

Assuming the validity of this model, there is need for a re-examination of those patients we rate as fully compliant as against those who, on occasion, act independently and, as a result, are judged inevitably by those who define the standards as non-compliant to some extent. This need, we believe, is compelling indeed when the label, "bad patient" is applied to those patients who desire to exercise their rights as patients to be well informed and when, Shelly Taylor (1979) reports ironically, that though a minority, their numbers are substantial enough to constitute a major medical problem!

In essence, we need to reevaluate the philosophical assumptions underlying our expectations and required standards for patients' behavior and whether patient or staff shall be the source of the norms against which harmful deviation from that regimen is calibrated.

The discussion in the preceding pages was intended to reflect two aspects of the great complexity of the issue of staff bias.

The issue raised in the section on "What Determines a Staff's View of Compliance?" concerns one important aspect of staff bias which cuts across many other dimensions of the problem discussed here, namely, bias operating in the judgment process, leading staff to label one patient as compliant and another as noncompliant. Also addressed in the present section is "Staff Bias as the Wrong Criterion." Such criterion problems impose themselves on studies of staff bias in a variety of ways. Problems with the criterion measure of compliance may be the reason for (1) statistics of such alarming proportions on the extent of the problem of noncompliance, as well as (2) some of the misguided research efforts wherein we strive to develop more and more elaborate methodological attempts to answer the wrong questions. Beyond these implications for the accuracy of demographics and experimental design of future research lies the question of the soundness of the criterion from a more philosophical standpoint, which, as noted, should lead us back to more careful consideration of our value systems.

REFERENCES

Alexander, L. The double-bind theory and hemodialysis. *Archives of General Psychiatry, 33,* 1353–1356, 1976.

Blank, J. Nurses' and patients' perception of the needs of the advanced cancer patient. Unpublished manuscript, Yale University School of Nursing, 1979.

Calland, C. H. Iatrogenic problems in end-stage renal failure. *New England Journal of Medicine, 287*(7), 334–336, 1972.

Czackes, J., & Kaplan De-Nour, A. *Chronic hemodialysis as a way of life.* New York: Brunner/Mazel, 1978.

Davidson, P. O. Therapeutic compliance. *Canadian Psychological Review, 17,* 247–259, 1976.

De-Nour, A. Prediction of adjustment to chronic hemodialysis. In N. B. Levy (Ed.), *Psychonephrology I: Psychological factors in hemodialysis and transplantation.* New York: Plenum, 1981.

De-Nour, A., & Czaczkes, J. W. Bias in assessment of patients on chronic dialysis. *Journal of Psychosomatic Research, 18,* 217–221, 1974.

DiMatteo, M. R., & DiNicola, D. O. *Achieving patient compliance.* New York: Pergamon, 1982.

Gerber, K. E. Staff vs. patient perception of life changes in hemodialysis patients. Paper presented at the annual meeting of the Western Dialysis and Transplant Society, 1980.

Gerber, K., Falke, R. & Ralidis, P. Social support and compliance to medical regimen in hemodialysis patients. Paper presented at the 64th Annual Meeting of the Western Psychological Association, Los Angeles, 1984.

Gerber, K. E., Nehemkis, A. M., Farberow, N. L., & Williams, J. Indirect self-destructive behavior in chronic hemodialysis patients. *Suicide and Life-Threatening Behavior, 11*(1), 31–42, 1981.

Gillmore, M. R., & Hill, C. T. Reactions to patients who complain of pain: Effects of ambiguous diagnosis. *Journal of Applied Social Psychology, 11,* 14–22, 1981.

Goldstein, A. P., & Shipman, W. G. Patient expectancies, symptom reduction and aspects of the initial psychotherapeutic interview. *Journal of Clinical Psychology, 17,* 129–133, 1961.

Hanson, R. W., & Franklin, M. R. Sexual loss in relation to other functional losses for spinal cord injured males. *Archives of Physical Medicine and Rehabilitation, 57,* 291–293, 1976.

Hyman, H. H., Cobb, W. J., Feldman, J. J., Hart, C. H., & Stember, C. H. *Interviewing in social research.* Chicago: University of Chicago Press, 1954.

Kasl, S. W. Issues in patient adherence to health care regimens. *Journal of Human Stress, 1,* 5–17, 1975.

Lorber, J. Good patients and problem patients: Conformity and deviance in a general hospital. *Journal of Health and Social Behavior, 16,* 213–225, 1975.

Masling, J. M. The influence of situational and interpersonal variables in projective testing. *Psychological Bulletin, 57,* 65–85, 1960.

Nehemkis, A. M., Gerber, K. E., & Charter, R. A. The cancer ward patient perceptions—staff misperceptions. *Psychotherapy and Psychosomatics, 41*(1), 42–47, 1984.

Nehemkis, A. M., & Groot, H. Indirect self-destructive behavior in spinal cord injury. In N. L. Farberow (Ed.), *The many faces of suicide: Indirect self-destructive behavior.* New York: McGraw-Hill, 1980.

Nehemkis, A. M., Stampp, M., & Amaral, P. Consultation issues on a cancer ward: The hidden agenda. *International Journal of Psychiatry in Medicine, 11*(4), 353–364, 1981–1982.

Orne, M. T. The nature of hypnosis: Artifact and essence. *Journal of Abnormal and Social Psychology, 58,* 277–299, 1959.

Pearson, L. Respondent. Coping with cancer: Confronting the diagnosis. In J. W. Cullen, B. H. Fox, & R. N. Isom (Eds.), *Cancer: The behavioral dimensions.* New York: Raven Press, 1976.

Rogers, B. The role of the psychiatrist in the renal dialysis unit. In R. Pasnau (Ed.), *Consultation—Liaison psychiatry,* New York: Grune and Stratton, 1975.

Rosenthal, R. On the social psychology of the psychological experiment: With particular reference to experimenter bias. Paper presented at the annual meetings of the American Psychological Association, New York, 1961.

Ross, L. The intuitive psychologist and his shortcomings: Distortions in the attribution process. In L. Berkowitz (Ed.), *Advances in experimental social psychology* (Vo. 10). New York: Academic Press, 1977.

Spradlin, W. W., & Porterfield, P. B. Patient compliance from a systems perspective. In D. J. Withersty, J. M. Stevenson, & R. H. Waldman (Eds.), *Communication and compliance in a hospital setting.* Springfield, IL: Charles C Thomas, 1980.

Stimson, G. V. Obeying doctor's orders: A view from the other side. *Social Science and Medicine, 8,* 97–104, 1974.

Stoner, J. A. F. A comparison of individual and group decisions involving risk. Unpublished master's thesis, M.I.T., 1961.

Straight, M. *After long silence.* New York: Norton, 1983.

Tagliacozzo, D. L., & Mauksch, H. O. The patient's view of the patient's role. In E. G. Jaco (Ed.), *Patients, physicians, and illness* (2nd ed.). New York: Free Press, 1972.

Taylor, S. E. Hospital patient behavior: Reactance, helplessness, or control? *Journal of Social Issues, 35*(1), 156–184, 1979.

Trillin, A. S. Of dragons and garden peas: A cancer patient talks to doctors. *New England Journal of Medicine, 304*(12), 699–701, 1981.

Turk, D., Meichenbaum, D., & Genest, M. *Pain and Behavioral Medicine.* New York: Guilford, 1983.

Wallach, M. A., & Kogan, N. The roles of information, discussion, and consensus in group risk taking. *Journal of Experimental Social Psychology,* *1,* 1–19, 1965.

Wallach, M. A., Kogan, N., & Bem, D. J. Diffusion of responsibility and level of risk taking in groups. *Journal of Abnormal and Social Psychology,* *68,* 263–274, 1964.

Weisman, A. D. *Coping with cancer.* New York: McGraw-Hill, 1979.

White, R. W. Strategies of adaptation: An attempt at systematic description. In G. V. Coelho, D. A. Hanburg, & J. E. Adams (Eds.). *Coping and Adaptation.* New York: Basic Books, 1974.

Wright, M. H., & Nehemkis, A. M. Functional use of secondary cancer symptomatology, *International Journal of Psychiatry in Medicine. 13*(4), 267–275, 1983–1984.

Yalom, I. *Existential psychotherapy,* New York: Basic Books, 1980.

Yeargan, L., & Nehemkis, A. M. The cancer ward: Scapegoating revisited. *Death Education, 7,* 1–7, 1983.

9

Physician-Patient Communication and Compliance

Richard W. Hanson

Recent efforts to understand the problem of noncompliance have focused increasingly on the interaction between the physician or other health care provider and the patient (DiMatteo & DiNicola, 1982; Kasl, 1975; Stone, 1979; Svarstad, 1976). In fact, the empirical investigation of patient–physician interactions is only beginning to receive attention (see review by Pendleton, 1983). Some investigations have involved process analyses of the verbal content of the interaction (e.g. Stiles, Putnam, Wolf, & James, 1979) or the nonverbal, affective dimensions of the interaction (e.g. Hall, Roter, & Rand, 1981). Other investigations have explored the relationship between process variables and outcome variables.

Pendleton (1983) suggests that outcomes can be immediate, intermediate, or long-term. One immediate outcome that has been studied extensively is patient satisfaction with medical care. In spite of some methodological and theoretical problems in this literature (Locker & Dunt, 1978), one consistent finding is that the major source of patient dissatisfaction concerns the patient-physician relationship. Pendleton (1983) summarizes the findings by saying,

> .... satisfaction of the patient is more likely when the doctor discovers and deals with the patient's concerns and expectations; when the doctor's manner communicates warmth, interest and concern about the patient; when the doctor volunteers a lot of information and explains things to the patient in terms that are understood. (p. 39)

Another important immediate outcome of the interaction is the patient's memory of the physician's instructions. Closely related to these immediate outcomes is compliance, the major immediate outcome variable mentioned by Pendleton (1983). Dissatisfaction with the interaction, communication problems, and failure to remember or to understand what they have been told are major sources of patient noncompliance with treatment recommendations. The communication of information and its relation to compliance will be discussed in greater length below.

A major long-term outcome of patient–physician interactions is ideally an improvement in the patient's health. However, more realistic outcomes for many chronic conditions may concern stabilization of the patient's condition and prevention of further deterioration or premature death. If the physician's treatment recommendations are indeed efficacious, one could presume that compliance with those recommendations will have a beneficient effect on the patient's health.

Following a section on the communication of information, we will consider other aspects of the physician–patient relationship and their effects on compliance. In particular, we will discuss means by which the physician can influence or persuade the patient to comply with treatment recommendations.

COMMUNICATION OF INFORMATION

An essential component of the patient–physician interaction is communication of information. Patients must accurately report information regarding their symptoms in order to assist the physician in making the correct diagnosis. In evaluating the efficacy of a therapeutic regimen, patients must report the manner or degree to which they have actually followed the presented regimen. The physician, on the other hand, must convey information to the patient regarding the results of diagnostic procedures, diagnosis, prognosis, and the treatment regimen. Information regarding the treatment regimen should include the rationale for a given procedure, the treatment options available, and the specific behaviors required by the patient in order to carry out the treatment regimen.

Thus, both patient and physician share responsibility for this exchange of information. However, Haney and Colson (1980) have argued that the greater responsibility in this interchange lies with the physician and that it is the ethical responsibility of the physician to learn the necessary communication skills to adequately convey information to the patient. Such communication skills involve more than simply conveying verbal information. Rather, attention must also be given to nonverbal aspects of communication as well as understanding the psychological, social, cultural, and situational variables that either facilitate or impede the communication process. Haney and Colson (1980) further argue that the acquisition of communication skills should be a component of formal medical education rather than left to chance acquisition through clinical experience.

With regard to compliance, it is obvious that patients cannot be expected to fully and accurately follow through on treatment recommendations unless they understand and remember the physician's instructions. Several studies have examined the degree to which patients understand and remember what the physicians told them (see reviews by Ley, 1982; 1983). For example, Joyce et al. (1969) interviewed a group of patients attending an outpatient medical clinic either immediately after the visit or after a delay of one to four weeks. These investigators found that patients were able to report an average of slightly less than half of the total items of information that they had been given irrespective of when they were interviewed. Although there were differences in the types of information retained, patients were able to recall less than half of the instructions regarding their treatment regimen.

A number of factors have been identified which may contribute toward physician–patient communication problems. These factors can be arbitrarily divided into physician variables, patient variables, and interactional variables.

PHYSICIAN VARIABLES

First of all, it is unreasonable to expect a patient to understand what behaviors are required unless the physician spends an adequate amount of time explaining the purpose and nature of the treatment regimen. One investigator found that in patient-physician encounters, which lasted an average of 20 minutes, only about one and a half minutes were spent in the transmission of information from the physician to the patient (Waitzkin & Stoeckle, 1976; Waitzkin, 1979). It was also found that physicians consistently overestimated the amount of time spent in giving information to patients and frequently underestimated the patient's desire for information. In relating time spent with physicians and compliance, Geertsen, Gray, and Ward (1973) found that the patient's perception of the amount of time spent with physicians was more important than the absolute amount of time. That is, patients who felt that their physician spent an inadequate amount of time with them were less likely to comply.

In addition to dissatisfaction with the amount of time their physicians spend with them, several studies have looked at patient's dissatisfaction with the communication of information. In Ley's (1982) review of such studies, he found considerable variability in dissatisfaction (range of 8 to 65 percent) with a median of about 36 percent. Direct observation or review of physician consultation transcripts has also suggested that patients are often given insufficient information regarding their treatment regimen (Svarstad, 1976).

Another important issue is the degree to which the physician conveys information in terms that the patient can understand. Although patients may be impressed by physician's use of medical jargon, they can hardly be expected to comply if they fail to understand what they are being asked to do. In an early study of medical vocabulary knowledge among hospital patients, Samora, Saunders, and Larson (1961) found that many patients either misunderstood or completely failed to understand many commonly used medical terms. This was especially evident among patients with lower education or who were of an ethnic group. Ley and his colleagues (see Ley, 1982) have found that many patients report that they did not understand the information presented. For example, one of his studies found that 43% of patients did not understand information regarding their treatment regimen.

In conclusion, it has been found that noncompliance may

result when physicians spend too little time with their patients, fail to communicate a sufficient amount of information, and do so in terms that the patient is not able to understand.

PATIENT VARIABLES

Several studies have suggested that patients simply forget much of what the physician tells them. Cassata (1978) summarized the physician–patient communication research as it relates to patient recall of information. The major conclusions are as follows:

1. Patients forget much of what the doctor tells them.
2. Instruction and advice are more likely to be forgotten than other types of information.
3. The more a patient is told, the greater the portion he or she will forget.
4. Patients will remember (a) what they are told first, and (b) what they consider most important.
5. Intelligent patients do not remember more than less intelligent patients.
6. Older patients remember just as much as younger ones.
7. Moderately anxious patients recall more of what they are told than highly anxious patients or patients who are not anxious.
8. The more medical knowledge a patient has, the more he or she will recall.
9. If the patient writes down what the doctor says, he or she will remember it just as well as if he or she merely hears it.

Communication of Information in Chronic Conditions

Much of the communication literature showing that patients frequently forget or misunderstand the information conveyed by their physicians is based on patients' first visits for a particular illness or on visits for acute conditions. Thus, it may be hypothesized that retention and understanding of information improves with repeated physician contacts as required by many chronic conditions. In reviewing the few relevant studies, Ley (1982) concludes that patient knowledge is better after repeated visits, but not that much better.

An even more significant issue related to chronic conditions is whether the patient remains in treatment. Baekeland and Lundwall (1975) provide a comprehensive review of the factors associated with dropping out of treatment. With regard to chronic medical conditions (such as hypertention), one factor associated with drop-out is poor instruction regarding the potential dangers of the condition as well as the importance of remaining in treatment. Another important factor is the degree of congruence between provider and patient ideas regarding the goals and methods of treatment.

INTERACTIONAL VARIABLES

Baekeland and Lundwall (1975) reviewed six studies, all of which found that discrepant therapist–patient treatment expectations were associated with dropping out of treatment. Although these studies focused on individual psychotherapy, the authors suggested that poorly informed patients who either fail to understand or disagree with the rationale are likely to drop out of other forms of treatment as well.

Other physician–patient discrepancies which may contribute to communication problems include differences in social status, education, and ethnic background. Such discrepancies may influence the amount of information which the physician assumes the patient desires and can understand. This is especially a problem since physicians generally tend to underestimate the comprehension level of their patients (Segall & Roberts, 1980). Pratt, Seligman, and Reader (1957) found that when physicians underestimated patient knowledge they also spent less time attempting to explain things to the patient.

Finally, the nature of the physician–patient interaction may significantly affect the communication process. For example, physicians who adopt a more formal, authoritarian role may intimidate passive, unassertive patients and prevent such patients from asking for additional or clarifying information.

Content of Information

In addition to examining the communication of information to patients, it is important to consider what types of information are most related to subsequent compliance. Although ideally the patient should be given information regarding the disease itself (e.g., diagnosis, etiology, severity or prognosis), evidence regarding the relationship between such knowledge and compliance is equivocal (Haynes, 1976). For example, Gordis, Markowitz, and Lillenfield (1969), Vincent (1971), and Weintraub, Au, and Lasagna (1973), and Bergman and Werner (1963) found no relationship between such knowledge and compliance. In addition, attempts to improve compliance by providing more information about the disease have occasionally met with failure (Sackett et al., 1975; Tagliacozzo, Luskin, Lashof, & Ima, 1974).

Nevertheless, as Masur (1981) points out, these negative results should be interpreted with caution. First, formal knowledge of the disease may not be as important as the patient's interpretation and subjective evaluation of such knowledge. Second, knowledge of the disease is not a unitary and easily quantifiable variable. Some types of information regarding the illness may be more important than others. For example, it may be more important that the patient understands the potential of hypertension than it is for him to understand the etiology of this disease. Third, one should not use compliance as the sole criteria on which to base patient education. Communication of information regarding the patient's disease may also contribute toward a healthy physician–patient collaborative relationship in which the patient assumes a more active role.

In addition to information regarding the disease itself, the other significant type of information concerns the treatment regimen itself. This may include the rationale for the regimen, the specific patient behavior required, and the possible consequences of failure to follow the regimen. Some of the studies mentioned above failed to find a relationship between knowledge of the treatment rationale and compliance (e.g. Weintraub, et al. 1973).

However, once again these findings should not be interpreted as indications that information regarding the rationale is not important. Formal knowledge of the rationale may not be as important as the patient's subjective interpretation and evaluation of the rationale. As Leventhal (1982) points out, a physician's presentation of information regarding the illness or treatment rationale may not be as important in itself as the degree to which such information corresponds with the patient's private theories about the illness and what should be done about it.

Information regarding the specific patient behaviors required in order to follow a given regimen is obviously the *sine qua non* for compliance. Such information is related to the type, or complexity, of medical recommendation given. A recommendation to stop smoking cigarettes is relatively clear and straightforward. The fact that many patients fail to comply with this recommendation is not likely due to their failure to know what they should do. On the other hand, multiple medication regimens tend to be more complicated. The patient must know what medications are to be taken, the number of pills or dose to be taken at each time, the frequency or timing of the medications, the mode and duration of medication usage. This requires clear, specific, and detailed instructions. Written prescriptions and subsequent prescription labels frequently do not include all this information (Boyd et al., 1974). Thus, it is necessary for the physician to spend the necessary time explaining such details to the patient and supplementing this with detailed written information or medication calendars. Ley (1982) also suggests that the patient's recall of information will be enhanced if the physician uses explicit categorization of material, simplified instructions, repetition by both physician and patient (e.g., asking the patient to restate the information given), and use of specific rather than general statements of advice.

THE PHYSICIANS INFLUENCE ON PATIENT COMPLIANCE

Presumably when there is ideal physician-patient communication of information, many patients will comply with their treatment instructions. At the same time, it is clear that some patients fail to comply even when there is a perfect exchange of information and the patient fully understands the nature and rationale of the treatment regimen. Thus, when patients fail to comply for reasons other than inadequate knowledge and comprehension, the physician may have to employ other strategies to improve compliance.

Before discussing these other strategies, it must be emphasized that a thorough assessment of the patient's compliance is necessary. First, it is necessary to determine whether the patient actually is noncompliant. Second, if the patient is noncompliant, it is important to determine whether it is due to inadequate knowledge and comprehension of the treatment regimen. Third, assuming the noncompliant patient has adequate knowledge, one must look for other factors contributing to the problem.

Assessing Compliance

One major implication of the compliance literature is that physicians cannot afford to simply take compliance for granted (Matthews & Hingson, 1977). Although assessing whether or not a given patient is compliant is an essential aspect of medical care, it is unfortunately often neglected by physicians. When treating chronic conditions, physicians do routinely monitor target physical symptoms. However, changes in symptomatology do not necessarily reflect degree of compliance. For example, consider a hypertensive patient being treated with medication. Although, it is often assumed that proper medication will reduce blood pressure, changes in measured blood pressure may or may not reflect actual compliance. Consequently, when a particular patient's blood pressure does not lower to acceptable levels, it may mean that either the patient is noncompliant or the medication may be ineffective. Since many physicians tend to overestimate their patients' compliance (Davis, 1966) and fail to directly monitor compliance, the physician in this case may erroneously assume that the medication is ineffective and thus prescribe a more powerful antihypertensive agent, when in fact the original medication may be sufficient if the patient was fully compliant. Thus, it is essential for the physician to determine the extent to which a patient is actually following a given treatment in order to assess the utility of that treatment.

In addition to the failure of many physicians to directly

assess patient compliance, it has been noted that patients often fail to report spontaneously their noncompliance and some may even deliberately distort the truth (DiMatteo & DiNicola, 1982). Although surreptitious compliance assessment techniques have been suggested for research purposes (e.g., pill counts, urine or blood assays, questioning family members), their use in clinical situations may be contraindicated. Consequently, we would agree with the position that direct physician inquiries regarding a patient's compliance should be sufficient given an adequate physician–patient relationship. The nature of such a relationship will be discussed later. Finally, it should be pointed out that active physician monitoring of patient's compliance may, in itself, facilitate improved compliance (Svarstad, 1976).

Assessing Reasons for Noncompliance

In addition to assessing the degree of patient compliance, it is important to determine what factors are contributing to compliance problems. Although this assessment naturally follows when a patient is discovered to be noncompliant with a particular treatment, a more ideal approach would be to assess in advance potential barriers for carrying out the recommendation. Thus, rather than waiting for compliance problems to develop and then discover them upon follow-up evaluation, a physician would be wise to assess possible compliance problems at the time treatment recommendations are initially given.

First, it is essential to determine whether the patient understands what he is being asked to do. After ensuring that the patient does understand the regimen, other factors can be explored. For example, Matthews and Hingson (1977) suggest that a "compliance-oriented history" should include inquiries regarding beliefs about the illness itself as well as beliefs about the treatment plan. Assessing the latter is especially important and should include questions aimed at determining the extent to which the patient agrees to the plan (e.g., perceived efficacy) and factors that may interfere with the patient's ability to carry it out.

Related to this evaluation, is Ley's (1979) distinction between voluntary and involuntary noncompliance. Involuntarily noncompliant patients may fully understand and agree to follow a treatment regimen but have difficulty carrying it out because of memory lapses, difficulties in incorporating it into their daily routine, excessive cost of treatment, etc. Such patients can be assisted by such procedures as simplifying the regimen, tailoring the regimen to coincide with daily activities, and using various reminders such as medication calendars and mechanical aids (e.g., pill dispensers, calorie counters). The voluntary or intentionally noncompliant patient, on the other hand, may fully understand the regimen but disagrees with it, is ambivalent about it, or does not wish to make major habit changes (e.g., lose weight, stop smoking, start an exercise program). According to Ley (1979) such patients require the use of more persuasive techniques. Persuasion may be directed at altering the patient's erroneous beliefs about the illness or treatment plan or it can be used to enhance motivation to make the necessary effort to follow through on the recommendations.

Before resorting to more persuasive tactics, however, the physician should make an attempt to determine the patient's perceptions of the treatment regimen including its anticipated consequences. Hayes-Bautista (1976) suggests that many cases of noncompliance represent the patient's attempts to modify a treatment program that is considered inappropriate. Two forms of intentional modification are augmentation and diminishment. Augmentation occurs when the patient believes the treatment is nominally appropriate but is insufficient. Thus, the patient may attempt to augment the treatment by increasing the dosage of a prescribed medication (i.e., taking more of the drug than originally prescribed) or may add other treatments (e.g., use medication originally prescribed for someone else, use nonprescription drugs, use home remedies, etc.). The diminishment form of treatment modification occurs when the patient perceives the treatment as being overly adequate. Thus, he may reduce the prescribed dosage or frequency or eliminate a particular medication all together. Such patient-initiated modifications of the treatment regimen can be precluded altogether or kept to a minimum by thoroughly evaluating the patient's perception of the regimen at the time it is instituted and after it has been initiated.

Physician-Patient Relationship

The success of a thorough compliance assessment requires a physician–patient relationship that allows and encourages open discussion of compliance issues. Further, it has been asserted that the mere process of conducting such an assessment can contribute toward the establishment of a good relationship, which in turn can facilitate improved compliance (Matthews & Hingson, 1977). The assessment process can communicate to the patient that the physician is genuinely interested in the patient's own appraisal of the treatment regimen and also appreciates the difficulties that may be involved in carrying it out.

Several models of physician–patient relationships have been suggested. Szasz and Hollender (1956), for example, presented three models. The activity-passivity model, in which the physician assumes an authoritarian role while the patient remains totally passive and helpless, is appropriate in some emergency situations (e.g., the patient is unconscious). In the guidance-cooperation model the patient still turns power over to the physician but is expected to participate more actively in his or her care by cooperating with the physician's instructions. This model, which is clearly dominant in current medical care delivery, is probably most appropriate for patients with certain acute problems (e.g., infections). In the third model, called mutual-participation, the physician and patient share approximately equal power and work together in a more collaborative manner. This model, although rare in modern medical practice, is probably more appropriate in the treatment of most adults with chronic conditions or with the parents of children having chronic conditions.

Brody (1980) suggests that the physician can encourage mutual participation in clinical decision making by taking four steps. The first step involves the initial establishment of a conducive atmosphere or good working relationship by helping the patient feel valued and appreciated. This can be facilitated by asking the patient open-ended questions and by responding promptly to all questions. Thus, the physician communicates interest in the chronically ill patient rather than just the disease itself. In the second step, the physician attempts to determine the patient's goals and expectations for treatment. The third step involves educating the patient about the problem, discussing pros and cons of alternative evaluation and treatment approaches, and explaining the specific recommendations. This need not involve an in-depth technical discussion of the pathophysiology of the disease or biochemistry of various medications (which most patients do not need or desire anyway). Instead, the discussion should focus more on beliefs, attitudes, and decisions based on the patient's understanding of the seriousness of the problem, the expected benefits of treatment, and the associated costs (financial, side-effects, etc.) of the recommended action. The final step involves eliciting the patient's informed suggestions and preferences and negotiating any disagreements with the patient over the best course of action.

In other words, the development of a treatment program is a negotiated process in which both physician and patient are actively involved. This does not mean that physicians must abrogate their responsibility by placing the patient in a totally self-care situation (Brody, 1980). Furthermore, since it is likely that many patients prefer to turn decision-making authority over to the physician, it is not necessary to force patients to decide among various treatment options. What should be avoided is the traditional paternalistic attitude whereby the physician assumes in advance what the patient needs to know and thus makes no attempt to include the patient in the decision-making process out of fear of burdening the patient with too much information or too much responsibility.

Another aspect of the mutual participation process is the recognition that patients have the right to refuse any treatment believed not to be in their best interest. Likewise, physicians have the right to refuse any patient suggestions which are judged likely to result in more harm than good. Brody (1980) also suggests that this process requires physician flexibility in considering alternative courses of action. Such flexibility can be enhanced by physicians' attempts to understand the patients' internal frame of reference regarding the nature of the disease, its seriousness, and expected consequences of various courses of action.

In addition to exploring the patient's perceptions of the

treatment regimen, Stone (1979) points out that the physician should have sufficient knowledge of human behavior to anticipate problems in following certain treatment recommendations. For example, if any major habit or lifestyle changes are recommended, the physician would be wise to automatically anticipate problems in initiating such changes, and more importantly, in maintaining such changes once made. Furthermore, by anticipating and discussing compliance problems in advance, it is likely that patients will feel more comfortable in admitting compliance failures and problems at subsequent visits without feeling they will be censured or blamed by the physician.

Thus, a mutual participation relationship has several advantages in facilitating patient compliance. By allowing patients to participate in the treatment planning process, they will be more likely to continue in treatment (Eisenthal, Emery, Lazare, & Udin, 1979) and many problems in following the treatment regimen can be avoided. Also, this type of relationship facilitates the identification and resolution of compliance problems which may develop when the patient does try to follow the regimen. DiMatteo and DiNicola (1982), in their excellent book on compliance, also devote considerable attention to the patient–physician relationship and advocate a "contractual model" (another term for the mutual participation model) as the ideal model for medical care. According to these authors:

> In the negotiated mutual contract (explicitly written or verbally agreed to) between the practitioner and patient, both have given informed consent to the regimen. There is a no-fault attitude toward non-compliant behavior, and the responsibility for the outcome of treatment is mutual. This ideal practitioner–patient relationship encourages, indeed expects, compliance behavior. The contract preserves the ideals of freedom for both parties, mutual understanding and mutual responsibility .... In the contractual relationship, neither party "loses." Rather, both "win" when compliance occurs because compliance is a mutually satisfactory outcome. (pp. 262–263)

While arguing for a mutual participation model, it must be recognized that the approach by no means guarantees compliance. Furthermore, at this point the model is probably based as much upon values as it is upon empirical findings. Unfortunately, the limited empirical literature on the physician-patient relationship and compliance is somewhat inconsistent and contradictory (Stone, 1979). For example, Geersten et al. (1973) found better compliance among arthritic patients who perceived their physician as personal rather than businesslike. Likewise, Francis, Korsch, and Morris (1969) found that mothers of ill children were more compliant with physicians perceived as friendly as compared to businesslike. Davis and Eichhorn (1963), on the other hand, found that cardiac patients were more compliant with physicians perceived as formal and businesslike rather than informal or friendly. Williams, Martin, Hogan, Watkins, and Ellis (1967) also found better compliance among diabetic patients who perceived their physicians as authoritarian. Davis (1971) examined doctor–patient interactions using Bale's Interacting Process Analysis. Although no significant relationships were found between measured interactions and compliance on the first visit, an analysis of interaction patterns on return visits indicated that compliant patients were more likely to accept passively what the doctor told them and not express opinions on their diagnoses, regimen, or illness in general. However, patients who took the initiative in asking the doctor for his opinion or suggestions were also more compliant. These findings by Davis and Eichhorn (1963), Davis (1971), and Williams et al. (1967) do not correspond very well with the mutual participation or contractual model.

At the same time, it is apparent that research on the relationship between physician–patient interactions and compliance is in its infancy. Further, it is likely that such relationships are extremely complex and involve a large number of interacting variables. For example, Svarstad (1976) found that physician expressions of friendliness and receptivity toward the patient as well as the use of demanding, authoritarian instructions were not very predictive of compliance. However, both approaches were associated with increased compliance when accompanied by a high level of patient instruction.

One fairly consistent finding, however, is that patients' satisfaction with their physician interactions is associated with increased compliance or remaining in treatment (e.g. Francis et al., 1969; Kincey, Bradshaw, & Ley, 1975). Another issue which we would like to raise is whether patient compliance should be the sole or major criterion for determining the nature of the physician–patient relationship. For example, if it is found that patients are more compliant with demanding, authoritarian physicians, does this alone justify use of such approaches toward patients? In order to examine this more thoroughly, let us first consider a theoretical model of the various means by which physicians can influence or persuade patients to comply with their treatment plan.

Social Influence and Social Power

In order to attain a broader perspective on various means by which a physician can influence a patient to comply, it is useful to draw from the social psychological literature on social influence and social power. Social influence refers to changes in cognitions, attitudes, or behavior of a person (target) that are attributable to the actions of another person (influencing agent). The potential ability of the agent to exert such influence over a target is referred to as social power (French & Raven, 1959).

Six modes of social power have been described by Raven (1974). Coercive power stems from the ability of the influencing agent to mediate punishment for the target. Such power usually takes the form of some threat (e.g., "If you don't comply with my recommendations, I will refuse to treat you anymore").

Reward power stems from the ability to mediate rewards. Such rewards may be material; however, in medical care settings they are more likely to be personal (e.g., extra time, attention, and positive regard) or may refer to privileges (e.g., "If you lose 20 pounds, I won't require you to take x medication").

Legitimate power is based on the target's acceptance of a role relationship with the agent that obligates the target to comply (e.g., "I'm your doctor and I know what's best for you"). Closely related is expert power based on the agent's possession of superior knowledge (e.g., "I know all about x disease, and this is the way it must be treated"). The prevailing model of medical care relies considerably on legitimate and expert power as bases for influencing patients. When a patient consults a physician for a particular health problem, he is expected to transfer power and authority regarding that problem to the physician who is assumed to possess the knowledge and expertise to deal with the problem. Thus, when the physician informs the patient of the diagnosis and the recommended course of treatment, the patient is automatically expected to comply with such recommendations. When a patient does not comply, many physicians construe this as a challenge to their legitimate authority and expertise.

Another related and commonly used source of social power is informational power. In this case, power is based on the persuasiveness of the information communicated by the agent to the target (e.g., "These are the medical findings regarding your condition and they indicate that you must take x medication"). Information may be especially persuasive if it arouses fear in the patient (e.g., "If you don't take this medication, your condition will deteriorate and you may die"). There is a relatively large body of social psychological literature on fear-arousing communications and attitude or behavior change. Although there is ongoing debate regarding differing theoretical models, Sutton (1982) reached the following conclusion based on his literature review: "Increases in fear are consistently associated with increases in intentional and behavioral measures of acceptance" (p. 333). Furthermore, he found little evidence to support the fear-drive model which assumes a nonmonotonic (inverted U-shaped) relationship between the degree of fear arousal and acceptance. In other words, rather than high degrees of fear arousal, interfering with acceptance, the findings suggest more of a monotonic relationship. Of course fear-arousing communications rarely operate in isolation. Sutton (1982) also found that when individuals perceived the recommended action as being efficacious in reducing some danger, there is increased intention to adopt that action. Second, there is some evidence that providing specific instructions about how to perform the recommended action leads to increased likelihood of following the recommendation.

It should be noted, however, that not all studies reviewed assessed actual behavior changes. Thus, there is strong evidence that fear-arousing communications affect intention to follow recommendations; however, the evidence is less strong for actual change in behavior. Although there is evidence that intention to act is a good predictor of actual behavior (Ajzen & Fishbein, 1980), the correspondence is not perfect. Furthermore, it is likely that there is even less correspondence between initial intention and sustained behavior change. For example, a fear-arousing message regarding the consequences of obesity may often lead to an intention to lose weight and even temporary weight losses. However, it is doubtful whether this message will be sufficient to evoke sustained weight loss. In addition to assuring efficacy and providing specific instructions for the recommended action, DiMatteo and DiNicola (1982) recommend eliciting a verbal or written public commitment to comply as well as specific behavioral instructions rather than general ones (e.g., "eat only at mealtimes," rather than "lose weight").

Another danger of high fear-arousing communications is that they may eventually evoke competing defensive strategies to deal with the threat. For example, a patient may be informed that unless he terminates cigarette smoking, the condition being treated will worsen and eventually result in death. This fear-arousing message may lead to initial cessation of smoking; however, later relapses (a common occurrence with attempts at major habit change) may re-evoke the original fear. One defensive strategy for coping with this fear is to avoid the source of the threatening message—the physician. Hence, the patient may decide to drop out of treatment rather than face further threats or blame by the physician.

In summary, it appears that information that evokes high fear arousal may indeed lead to compliance. However, the compliance may be short lived and may lead to noncompliant defensive reactions to avoid the source of the communication.

Another problem with the types of social power discussed thus far is that when they do result in compliance, patients may attribute their compliance to external incentives rather than internalizing personal responsibility for, or control over, their actions. Ideally, physicians' use of social power should facilitate internal feelings of control and self-motivated compliance, especially when sustained behavior change is required as in chronic disorders (Kopel & Arkowitz, 1975).

In their discussion of various sources of social power, Rodin and Janis (1979) suggest that referent power is more conducive to an internalization of treatment recommendations. As originally defined by French and Raven (1959), referent power occurs when the target uses others as a frame of reference or standard for evaluating the target's behavior. In other words, the physician could mention other individuals whom the patient values and who are in a similar situation, as compliant models. However, Rodin and Janis (1979) suggest that the physician could become a source of referent power. Such power is developed when patients view their physicians as (1) being similar to themselves in beliefs, attitudes, and values, (2) having a benevolent, caring attitude toward them, and (3) accepting them as worthwhile individuals in spite of their apparent weaknesses and shortcomings. In short, the physician assumes the role of a significant reference person in the life of the patient. Physicians who have repeated contacts with chronic patients over time are especially well suited toward the development of this role. Referent power is not viewed in opposition to the other forms of social power. Rather, it is asserted that physicians who do rely on other types of power can enhance their effectiveness in facilitating compliance by developing and using referrent power.

The establishment and use of referrent power is discussed in three phases (Janis, 1983; Rodin & Janis, 1979). During the first phase, the physician or health care provider should encourage patient self-disclosure and then respond to these disclosures with acceptance, understanding, and unconditional positive regard. With regard to compliance, two types of patient self-disclosure should be encouraged. First, an attempt should be made to determine the patient's attitudes toward and expectations of the treatment regimen. This is necessary to determine whether compliance problems stem from the patient's lack of acceptance of the treatment regimen or doubts regarding its efficacy. Second, patients should be encouraged to disclose personal feelings, conflicts, weaknesses, etc., that may interfere with their ability to carry out the treatment recommendations.

During this process of encouraging and accepting patient self-disclosure, a cohesive, trusting therapeutic relationship is established enabling the physician to use referent power to facilitate compliance. This constitutes the second phase. In addition to the use of expert power, the practitioner can use referent power to persuade patients to accept the treatment recommendations, encourage or motivate them to make major lifestyle changes if indicated, reassure them of the efficacy of these actions, and assist them in coping with the difficulties and discomforts that may arise when they attempt to follow the recommendations.

Within this context, the use of information power, or statements regarding the necessity of following the regimen and negative consequences of not following it, is presented in a manner that is interpreted by the patient as caring concern rather than threat or coercion. Without establishment of referent power, these same statements may provoke high fear and subsequent compliance; however, the compliance may be short lived, and entirely externally motivated.

The third phase, according to Rodin and Janis (1979), is maintaining referent power in order to promote further internalization of treatment recommendations and to anticipate treatment termination. Treatment of many chronic conditions is terminated when the patient's condition becomes stabilized. Thus, the physician should prepare the patient for termination by reassuring the patient of continued positive regard, arranging for gradual rather than an abrupt termination (e.g., through telephone follow-up contacts) and leaving the door open for later contacts should the patient's condition change. In addition, the patient should be positively reinforced and given credit for changes made in order to increase feelings of self-efficacy and a sense of personal responsibility.

The Role of Other Health Care Providers

Throughout this chapter, emphasis has been placed on the role of the physician. Obviously, the physician has primary responsibility for the provision of medical care. However, many physicians may object to the recommendations presented because of time pressures. A full explanation of a patient's condition and treatment regimen, a thorough assessment and exploration of compliance issues with the patient, the establishment of a mutual participation relationship, and the development of referent power to influence that patient all may require considerable physician time. Since the focus of this volume is on chronic conditions, it has been assumed that the physician has repeated contacts with a patient over time thereby facilitating the utilization of our recommendations. Nevertheless, it still may be impractical for a busy physician to spend large amounts of time with each noncompliant or potentially noncompliant patient. Thus, it is unreasonable to expect physicians to be the sole providers involved in compliance issues. Patient education and detailed instruction regarding the treatment regimen can also be provided by nurses, physicians' assistants, pharmacists, dieticians, or other health care professionals routinely involved in the patient's care.

One general category of treatment recommendations which most likely requires assistance from other health care providers is lifestyle or habit change. Dietary changes, weight loss, smoking cessation, abstinence from alcohol, physical exercise programs, and stress management all require major habit changes or alteration in daily routine which are difficult to initiate and sustain. Although some individuals are able to make such changes on their own, others require assistance which is beyond the traditional scope of the physician. Nurses, dieticians, physical rehabilitation specialists, and psychologists may offer valuable assistance in these cases. Furthermore, patients can be referred to various community and commercial self-help programs involved in some of these specialties (e.g., smoking cessation, weight reduction, and exercise facilities).

Another recommendation that has been made is the establishment or designation of special compliance experts or compliance programs. Ulmer (1980), for example, recommends the establishment of a compliance team and a compliance specialist to deal with compliance issues in cancer patients. He suggests that this compliance specialist should have a particular interest in compliance and should be knowledgeable of the relevant literature. A psychologist or nurse are mentioned as the most likely candidates for this position. Also, in accord with this recommendation, Ulmer has established his own "noncompliance institute" which serves as a consultation service to physicians (Elsner, 1978). Noncompliant patients may also be referred directly to this noncompliance institute.

At this point we would question the necessity and utility of specially designated noncompliance experts or programs. Some patients may resent being labeled as noncompliant and thus in need of a special compliance expert. Such referrals may also undermine the mutual participation relationship. We would recommend that compliance issues be primarily addressed by those health professionals who are directly and routinely involved in the patient's care. If it becomes necessary to refer the patient to another professional, the referral should be a mutually agreed upon decision based upon the patient's difficulties in following a specific recommendation. For example, if a patient is not complying with instructions to stop smoking and it has been determined that the patient agrees with this recommendation but is having difficulty breaking the habit, the patient and physician may decide that the services of another professional trained in behavior change methods (e.g., a psychologist) may be needed. In this case, the explicit basis for referral would be assistance in smoking cessation rather than noncompliance.

THE LIMITS OF COMPLIANCE

A final issue which needs to be raised is whether compliance should be the final goal of patient response to medical care. Davidson (1982) reminds us that a review of the history of medicine clearly indicates that compliance is not a simple function of treatment efficacy. Many early, widely used treatment procedures are now considered either totally ineffective or even dangerous. A partial list of such techniques include purging, puking, poisoning, puncturing, cutting, cupping, blistering, bleeding, leeching, heating, freezing, sweating, and shocking (Shapiro & Morris, 1978). Thus, in some cases, noncompliance may have been necessary for survival. Consequently, Davidson (1982) suggests that we have an ethical responsibility to assure the efficacy of a given treatment before we set about increasing compliance to that treatment.

It has also been asserted that sometimes patients have valid reasons for not complying with prescribed medication, a situation referred to as "intelligent noncompliance" (Weintraub, 1976). One valid reason for noncompliance is the presence of dangerous side effects associated with toxic reactions to excess prescribed medication or interactions with other drugs. Other valid reasons may stem from diagnostic errors or use of inappropriate treatments. The point is, of course, that physicians do occasionally err in their prescribed treatment and that sometimes the patient knows best. Weintraub (1976) also suggests that in some chronic conditions, patients may have valid reasons for eventually discontinuing certain medications even though the physician continues to prescribe the medication out of fear of disturbing the status quo. He reminds physicians that "patients change, diseases run their course (even chronic conditions), other processes supervene—all of which may make therapy of the primary condition unnecessary." Once again it is asserted that physicians must do a better job of assessing the degree of noncompliance along with the patient's reasons in order to maximize the benefits and decrease the negative effects of intelligent noncompliance.

A second issue that we have already raised concerns the methods used to increase compliance. Another way of stating this is to ask whether the end justifies the means. Are forceful, coercive, threatening, and high fear-arousing techniques justified even when they do elicit patient compliance? Such techniques have been questioned because of the tendency for patients to attribute their compliant behavior to external factors rather than internally generated factors (Davidson, 1982; Rodin & Janis, 1979). Such externally attributed behavior changes are also less likely to be maintained over time. Thus, Kopel and Arkowitz (1975) advocate using the least powerful reward or punishment techniques to elicit behavior changes. Less powerful techniques include social influence based on referrent power (Rodin & Janis, 1979) and use of self-management strategies including self-reinforcement, self-monitoring, behavioral contracts, and self-instructional training (Davidson, 1982).

A final issue involves the recognition that no matter what approach or procedures are used, some patients will not be compliant. The following case illustrates this point:

Dr. S., a 48-year-old successful orthopedic surgeon discovered that he has severe essential hypertension. Consequently, he consulted an older, trusted, and highly respected colleague who was considered a major expert in this disease. This colleague carefully and thoroughly evaluated Dr. S., provided him with complete and detailed information regarding the findings, and reminded him of the basic facts of hypertension and the current state of the art concerning the treatment of this disorder. The colleague then placed Dr. S. on a particular antihypertensive medication regimen, a low-salt diet, and strongly recommended that he lose approximately 30 pounds of body weight. Dr. S. thoroughly understood and agreed to this treatment regimen including its rationale. He then began taking his medication faithfully and carefully followed his diet. However, after a few weeks he began to forget to take his medication with increasing frequency because of his extremely busy and erratic work schedule and he neglected his diet because of his great fondness for eating. Later when he was reevaluated by his colleague, it was found that his blood pressure was still dangerously high. Dr. S. admitted that he had not been following his treatment regimen very consistently and together they explored some of the reasons why. The colleague then reminded Dr. S. of the importance of following the regimen, prescribed additional medication to facilitate weight loss, and recommended that he seek other professional assistance (e.g., a hypnotherapist) to help him stick to his diet. Dr. S. once again verbally agreed to these recommendations but later failed to follow through on the recommendation to seek other assistance for weight reduction because he was too busy. He also began taking his medication inconsistently.

In this case, the patient, who also happened to be a physician, had full and complete knowledge of his disorder, its risks, and the treatment regimen. The relationship he had with his physician-colleague was based on mutual power, respect, and trust. Nevertheless, he was still noncompliant presumably because he was unwilling to make necessary lifestyle modifications. What additional steps could or should the treating physician take to elicit compliance? It is suggested that there may be occasions in which the physician does "all the right things" in terms of communication of information, the establishment of a mutual participation relationship, and the use of social influence based on referent power and still fails to elicit full patient compliance. As in the case above, noncompliance may be unintentional (i.e., the patient initially intends to comply but doesn't or does it erratically). In other cases, noncompliance may be intentional (e.g., the patient does not fully agree to the treatment plan).

One question that might be raised is whether the physician should continue treating the persistently noncompliant patient. Jonsen (1979), in his discussion of the ethical issues in such situations, suggests that the physician first ask himself if he rightly understands and appreciates the patient's motives, life setting, and comprehension as well as his own efforts, skills, and strategies to facilitate compliance. If, after such an examination of conscience, the physician believes that he has done everything possible, he should next consider whether it is appropriate to shift from a curing to a caring mode of treatment. It has been recommended that health care providers shift to an explicit caring role with the terminally ill patient. Of course in such cases, the presumed basis for this shift is the judgment that medical interventions are no longer effective. But what about those cases in which it is assumed that intervention would be effective but, however, the patient fails to comply with the recommended intervention? Although it is very difficult for most physicians trained in a primarily technological approach in medicine to adopt a caring role, it could be argued that in some cases the provision of psychosocial support, acceptance, and understanding may be as efficacious as medication. Furthermore, Jonsen (1979) questions whether health should be considered a unique or singular goal. The desire to restore or maintain patient health should not compromise other valid human goals such as the preservation of freedom, human dignity, and self-determination. If the fully informed patient decides that compliance with a particular treatment interferes with these other human goals, should we not respect this decision? Some of the same issues raised in discussions regarding the use of heroic measures to prolong life may apply. Should prolongation of life take precedence over quality of life? Clearly there are no simple answers to such dilemmas.

Another question regarding the shift from a curing to a caring mode with noncompliant patients relates to limits on physicians' time and medical resources (Jonsen, 1979). The physician may justifiably decide that his diagnostic and therapeutic skills may be better used elsewhere (i.e., with more compliant patients). If in such cases the physician deems it necessary to terminate a relationship with a noncompliant patient, some ethical guidelines should be adhered to. First, the physician should avoid abrupt, unilateral decisions to discontinue care. An attempt should be made to openly discuss the issue with the patient and explore alternative sources of medical or even nonmedical care. Referral to another health care professional may be indicated. Or in some cases the patient may decide to seek the services of a quasi-medical provider whom the physician considers as offering useless treatment. For example, some patients with cancer may prefer alternate, unconventional treatment approaches rather than submit to the discomforts of more traditional cancer regimens. In such cases, the physician may feel an ethical responsibility to share with the patient his reservations regarding such approaches; however, ultimately the patient should have the right to make such choices. Of course the issue is more complex when the patient is a child and the parents make the decision to seek unconventional treatment. Nonetheless, physicians would be wise to recognize the limits of technological medicine and realize that alternative, unconventional healers do have something valuable to offer (e.g., hope, encouragement, and social support) even if their specific methods lack scientific validity. The literature on placebo effects clearly indicates that nonspecific factors such as expectation can elicit positive therapeutic changes even to the point of physiological changes (Frank, 1973; Shapiro & Morris, 1978).

Thus, it is our belief that compliance should not necessarily be the final or singular goal of patient response to medical care. In some cases the patient may have valid reasons for noncompliance. In other cases the patient may intentionally or unintentionally fail to comply with resulting adverse effects on health, in spite of our best efforts. Rather than spending all of our effort on finding or utilizing powerful behavior modification technologies to control or manipulate patients to comply, more effort should be directed in the clinical situation to listen to patients and to understand noncompliance from the patient's frame of reference. If after doing everything possible within the context of a contractual or mutual-participation relationship, and the patient continues not to comply, then the patient's decision should be respected. The physician then must decide whether to shift to a caring mode, negotiate a gradual termination of treatment, or refer the patient to someone else.

CONCLUSION

The interaction between physician and patient plays a crucial role in determining the degree to which patients comply with their treatment program. First of all, patients must be given adequate information regarding the regimen and its rationale in order to properly carry out their physician's instructions. Communication of information is not a one-way process. Rather, the physicial should also elicit feedback from the patient to make sure that he understands the instructions and at least intends to carry them out. Problems with the patient's later recollection of instructions should be anticipated in advance, especially with more complicated medication or dietary regimens. An attempt should be made to keep the regimen as simple as possible and, if necessary, supplement verbal instructions with clear written instructions and prompts (e.g., medication calendars).

Most important, however, is the establishment of a mutually collaborative or contractual relationship which allows for an open and honest two-way interaction. In such a relationship, the patient's opinions, beliefs, and conceptualization of the disease and treatment expectations are taken into account. Such a relationship has several advantages. First, it may prevent compliance problems from arising in the first place. Second, it facilitates the early identification of compliance problems if and when they do occur. Third, it allows the physician to assess accurately the reasons for specific noncompliant behaviors. And finally, it enables the physician to more effectively influence the patient, using referent power, to make the necessary effort to follow the treatment instructions. Thus, rather than viewing noncompliance as a power struggle between physician and patient, akin to a parent's efforts to manage a rebellious child, compliance is a shared, mutually negotiated endeavor.

Finally, it must be accepted that some patients may continue to be noncompliant in spite of our best efforts. A mutual-participatory patient–physician relationship based on mutual respect can then allow such patients to retain their freedom and right to self-determination by recognizing that health is only one of several valid human goals.

BIBLIOGRAPHY

Ajzen, I., & Fishbein, M. *Understanding attitudes and predicting social behavior.* Englewood Cliffs, NJ: Prentice-Hall, 1980.

Baekeland, F., & Lundwall, L. Dropping out of treatment: A critical review. *Psychological Bulletin, 82,* 738-783, 1975.

Becker, M. H. (Ed.) *The health belief model and personal health behavior.* Thorofare, NJ: Charles B. Slack, 1974.

Becker, M. H., & Maiman, L. A. Sociobehavioral determinants of compliance with health and medical care recommendations. *Medical Care, 13,* 10-24, 1975.

Becker, M. H., & Maiman, L. A. Strategies for enhancing patient compliance. *Journal of Community Health, 6,* 113-135, 1980.

Becker, M. H., Maiman, L. A., Kirscht, J. P., Haefner, D. P., & Drachman, R. H. The health belief model and prediction of dietary compliance: A field experiment. *Journal of Health and Social Behavior, 18,* 348-366, 1977

Becker, M. H., Maiman, L. A., Kirscht, J. P. Haefner, D. P., Drachman, R. H., & Taylor, D. W. Patient perceptions and compliance: Recent studies of the health belief model. In R. B. Haynes, D. W. Taylor, & D. L. Sackett (Eds.), *Compliance in health care.* Baltimore: Johns Hopkins University Press, 1979.

Becker, M. H., Radius, S. M., Rosenstack, L. M., Drachman, R. H., Schuberth, K. C., & Teets, K. C. Compliance with a medical regimen for asthma: A test of the health belief model. *Public Health Reports, 93,* 268-277, 1978.

Bergman, A. B., & Werner, R. J. Failure of children to receive penicillin by mouth. *New England Journal of Medicine, 268,* 1334-1338, 1963.

Boyd, J. R., Covington, R. R., Stanaszek, W. F., & Coussons, R. T. Drug defaulting, Part II: Analysis of noncompliance patterns. *American Journal of Hospital Pharmacology, 31,* 485-491, 1974.

Brody, D. S. The patient's role in clinical decision making. *Annals of Internal Medicine, 93,* 718-722, 1980.

Cassata, D. M. Health communication theory and research: An overview of the communication specialist interface. In B. D. Ruben (Ed.), *Communication yearbook 2.* New Brunswick, NJ: Transaction Books, 1978.

Davidson, P. O. Issues in patient compliance. In T. Millon, C. Green, & R. Meagher (Eds.), *Handbook of clinical health psychology.* New York: Prenum Press, 1982.

Davis, M. S. Variations in patients' compliance with doctors' orders: Analysis of congruence between survey responses and results of empirical investigations. *Journal of Medical Education, 41,* 1037-1048, 1966.

Davis, M. S. Variation in patients' compliance with doctors' orders: Medical practice and doctor-patient interaction. *Psychiatry in Medicine, 2,* 31-54, 1971.

Davis, M. S., & Eichhorn, R. L. Compliance with medical regimens: A panel study. *Journal of Health and Human Behavior, 4,* 240-249, 1963.

DiMatteo, M. R., & DiNicola, D. D. *Achieving patient compliance: The psychology of the medical practitioner's role.* New York: Pergamon Press, 1982.

Dunbar, J. M., & Agras, W. S. Compliance with medical instructions. In J. H. Ferguson & C. B. Taylor (Eds.), *The comprehensive handbook of behavioral medicine.* Vol. 3. (pp. 115-145). Jamaica, NY: Spectrum Publications, 1980.

Dunbar, J. M., & Stunkard, A. J. Adherence to diet and drug regimen. In R. Levy, B. Rifkind, B. Dennis, & N. Ernst (Eds.), *Nutrition, lipids and coronary in heart disease.* (pp. 391-423). New York: Raven Press, 1979.

Eisenthal, S., Emery, R., Lazare, A., & Udin, H. "Adherence" and the negotiated approach to patienthood. *Archives of General Psychiatry, 36,* 393-398, 1979.

Elsner, R. H. Patient compliance as important as physician competence: *LACMA physician-bulletin of the Los Angeles County Medical Association,* October 5, 1978.

Francis, V., Korsch, B. M., & Morris, M. J. Gaps in doctor-patient communication. *New England Journal of Medicine, 280,* 535-540, 1969.

Frank, J. D. *Pursuasion and healings.* Baltimore: Johns Hopkins University Press, 1973.

French, J. R. P., Sr, & Raven, B. H. The bases of social power. In D. Cartwright (Ed.), *Studies in social power.* (pp. 150-167). Ann Arbor, MI: Institute for Social Research, University of Michigan, 1959.

Geertsen, H. R., Gray, R. M., & Ward, J. R. Patient compliance within the context of medical care for arthritis. *Journal of Chronic Diseases, 26,* 689-698, 1973.

Gordis, L., Markowitz, M., & Lilienfield, A. M. Why patients don't follow medical advice: A study of children on long-term antistreptococcal prophylaxis. *Journal of Pediatrics, 75,* 957-968, 1969.

Hall, J. A., Roter, D. L., & Rand, C. S. Communication of affect between patient and physician. *Journal of Health and Social Behavior, 22,* 18-30, 1981.

Haney, C. A., & Colson, A. C. Ethical responsibility in physician-patient communication. *Ethics in Science and Medicine, 7,* 27-36, 1980.

Hartman, P. E., & Becker, M. H. Noncompliance with prescribed regimen among chronic hemodialysis patients. *Dialysis and Transplantation, 7,* 978-989, 1978.

Haynes-Bautista, D. E. Modifying the treatment: Patient compliance, patient control and medical care. *Social Science and Medicine, 10,* 233-238 1976.

Hayes, R. B. A critical review of the "determinants" of patient compliance with therapeutic regimens. In D. L. Sackett & R. B. Haynes (Eds.), *Compliance with therapeutic regiments.* Baltimore: Johns Hopkins University Press, 1976.

Haynes, R. B. Taylor, D. W., & Sackett, D. L. (Eds.), *Compliance in health care.* Baltimore: Johns Hopkins University Press, 1979.

Janis, I. L. The role of social support in adherence to stressful decisions. *American Psychologist, 38,* 143-160, 1983.

Jonsen, A. R. Ethical issues in compliance. In R. B. Haynes, D. W. Taylor, & D. L. Sackett (Eds.), *Compliance in health care.* Baltimore: Johns Hopkins University Press, 1979.

Joyce, C. R. B., Caple, G., Mason, M., Reynolds, E., & Mathews, J. A. Quantitative study of doctor-patient communication. *Quarterly Journal of Medicine, 38,* 183-194, 1969.

Kasl, S. V. The health belief model and behavior related to chronic illness. In M. H. Becker (Ed.), *The health belief model and personal health behavior.* (pp. 107-127). Thorofare, NJ: Charles B. Slac, 1974.

Kasl, S. V. Issues in patient adherence to health care regimens. *Journal of Human Stress, 1,* 5-17, 1975.

Kincey, J., Bradshaw, P., & Ley, P. Patients' satisfaction and reported acceptance of advice in general practice. *Journal of the Royal College of General Practitioners, 25,* 558-566, 1975.

Kirscht, J. P., & Rosenstock, I. M. Patient adherence to antihypertensive medical regimens. *Journal of Community Health, 3,* 115-124, 1977.

Kopel, S., & Arkowitz, H. The role of attribution and self-perception in behavior change: Implications for behavior therapy. *Genetic Psychology Monographs, 92,* 175-212, 1975.

Leventhal, H. Wrongheaded ideas about illness. *Psychology Today, 73,* 48-55, January 1982.

Ley, P. The psychology of compliance. In D. J. Oborne, M. M. Gruneberg, J. R. Eiser (Eds.), *Research in psychology and medicine, Vol. 2.* London: Academic Press, 1979.

Ley, P. Giving information to patients. In J. R. Eiser (Ed.), *Social Psychology and behavioral medicine.* New York: John Wiley, 1982.

Ley P. Patients' understanding and recall in clinical communication failure. In D. Pendleton & J. Hasler (Eds.), *Doctor-patient communication.* New York: Academic Press, 1983.

Locker, D., & Dunt, D. Theoretical and methodological issues in sociological studies of consumer satisfaction with medical care. *Social Science and Medicine, 12,* 283-292, 1978.

Masur, F. T. Adherence to health care regimens. In C. K. Prokop & L. A. Bradley (Eds.), *Medical psychology: Contributions to behavioral medicine.* New York: Academic Press, 1981.

Matthews, D., & Hingson, R. Improving patient compliance: A guide for physicians. *Medical Clinics of North America, 61,* 879-889, 1977.

Mischel, W. *Personality and assessment.* New York: John Wiley, 1968.

Ort, R. S., Ford, A. B., & Liske, R. E. The doctor-patient relationship as described by physicians and medical students. *Journal of Health and Human Behavior, 5,* 25-34, 1964.

Pendleton, D. Doctor-patient communication: A review. In D. Pendleton & J. Hasler (Eds.), *Doctor-patient communication.* New York: Academic Press, 1983.

Pratt, L., Seligmann, A., & Reader, G. Physicians' views on the level of medical information among patients. *American Journal of Public Health, 47,* 1277-1283, 1957.

Raven, B. H. The comparative analysis of power and influence. In J. T. Tedeschi (Ed.), *Perspectives on social power.* Chicago: Aldine, 1974.

Rodin, J., & Janis I. L. The social power of health-care practitioners as agents of change. *Journal of Social Issues, 35,* 60-81, 1979.

Sackett, D. L., Gibson, E. S., Taylor, D. W., Haynes, R. B., Hackett, B. C., Roberts, R. S., & Johnson, A. L. Randomized clinical trial of strategies for improving medication compliance in primary hypertension. *Lancet, 1,* 1205–1207, 1975.

Samora, J., Saunders, L., & Larson, R. Medical vocabulary knowledge among hospital patients. *Journal of Health and Human Behavior, 2,* 83–92, 1961.

Segall, A., & Roberts, L. W. A comparative analysis of physician estimates and levels of medical knowledge among patients. *Sociology of Health and Illness, 2,* 317–334, 1980.

Shapiro, A. K., & Morris, L. A. The placebo effect in medical and psychological therapies. In S. L. Garfield & A. E. Bergin (Eds.), *Handbook of psychotherapy and behavior change: An empirical analysis.* New York: John Wiley, 1978.

Stiles, W. B., Putnam, S. M., Wolf, M. H., & James, S. A. Verbal response mode profiles of patients and physicians in medical screening interviews. *Journal of Medical Education, 54,* 81–89, 1979.

Stone, G. C. Patient compliance and the role of the expert. *Journal of Social Issues, 35,* 34–59, 1979.

Sutton, S. R. Fear-arousing communications: A critical examination of theory and research. In J. R. Eiser (Ed.), *Social psychology and behavioral medicine.* New York: John Wiley, 1982.

Svarstad, B. L. Physician-patient communication and patient conformity with medical advice. In D. Mechanic (Ed.), *The growth of bureaucratic medicine: An inquiry into the dynamics of patient behavior and the organization of medical care.* New York: John Wiley, 1976.

Szasz, T. S., & Hollender, M. H. A contribution to the philosophy of medicine: The basic models of the doctor–patient relationship. *Archives of Internal Medicine, 97,* 585–592, 1956.

Tagliacozzo, D. M., Luskin, D. B., Lashof, J. C., & Ima, K. Nurse intervention and patient behavior: An experimental study. *American Journal of Public Health, 64,* 596–603, 1974.

Ulmer, R. A. *Noncompliance problems of cancer patients and their resolution.* Unpublished manuscript, Martin Luther King, Jr. General Hospital, 1980.

Vincint, P. Factors influencing patient noncompliance: A theoretical approach. *Nursing Research, 20,* 509–516, 1971.

Waitzkin, H. Medicine, superstructure and micropolitics. *Social Science and Medicine, 13,* 601–609, 1979.

Waitzkin, H., & Stoeckle, J.D. Information control and the micropolitics of health care: Summary of an ongoing research project. *Social Science and Medicine, 10,* 263–276, 1976.

Weintraub, M. Intelligent noncompliance and capricious compliance. In L. Lasagna (Ed.), *Patient compliance,* Mt. Kisco, NY: Futura, 1976.

Weintraub, M., Au, W., & Lasagna, L. Compliance as a determinant of serum digoxin concentration. *Journal of the American Medical Association, 224,* 481–485, 1973.

Williams, T. F., Martin, D., Hogan, M., Watkins, J., & Ellis, E. The clinical picture of diabetic control, studied in four settings. *American Journal of Public Health, 57,* 441–451, 1967.

10

How Society Contributes
to Noncompliance

Carol Cummings
Alexis M. Nehemkis

INTRODUCTION

Medical noncompliance takes many forms, from failure to seek
health care to fraudulent and self-inflicted injuries. As earlier
chapters have shown, the psychological meaning of such behavior
is as complex and various as its manifestations. Like other human
behavior, it is multidetermined, making it difficult to separate
the purely personal components of noncompliance from those
aspects which can be traced to the policies and structure of the
modern health care system.

The costs of noncompliance are enormous. They include all
the forms of compensation paid for illnesses and disabilities that
are caused by noncompliance as well as lost productivity and the
perpetuation of preventable diseases and chronic disorders. One
has only to consider the bills for the medical treatment of alcoholics who continue to drink, or smokers who die from lung
cancer, and all the others whose illnesses are caused or exacerbated
by habits they are unable to control. These are costs that could,
in theory, be reduced to monetary figures.

There are other results of noncompliance which cannot be
expressed in dollars but may be equally detrimental to society
in the long run. What are the intangible consequences to the
larger community when increasing numbers of its members are
willing to accept a nonproductive role by remaining unnecessarily
disabled?

With the understanding that noncompliance is never simple to explain, this chapter will focus on some of the ways in which social problems become medical problems. It will also examine how social pressures, by fostering noncompliance, can magnify the damage that is caused by illness. Finally, the question of values will arise. That is, in some situations it is a matter of one's values to determine when failure to comply with doctor's orders is rational or irrational. Depending upon one's point of view, non-compliance can be viewed as self-destructive, a sign of maturity and responsibility, or even a practical economic decision.

SOCIETY'S CONTRIBUTIONS TO NONCOMPLIANCE

There are shortcomings in our society, and especially in our health care system, that foster and perpetuate noncompliance. Among these are legal shackles, the structure of our health care institutions, and a compensation system which, combined with employer reluctance to rehire injured workers, certainly removes the financial incentive to get well in a hurry.

Factors Impeding Treatment of the Chronically Ill

The skid rows of our major cities are the homes of disheveled, muttering "shopping bag ladies" with swollen ankles and sores on their bodies. Hidden away in sleazy hotels are those who are so frightened and withdrawn that they seldom leave their rooms. Many of these pathetic men and women are chronic schizophrenics, too disordered to comply with a treatment program of visits to a mental health center and regular ingestion of appropriate antipsychotic medications.

They are helpless victims of two trends in mental health administration. The first is the closing of the big state mental hospitals, ostensibly to offer better care by restoring the mentally ill to their old communities where they are supposed to be followed by community mental health centers. Unfortunately, the funding and staffing of these centers has been greatly reduced in recent years. The second trend was to restrict the ability of the mental health professionals to detain or treat psychotic persons involuntarily unless they are a danger to themselves or others. Even in those cases, there are usually very strict time limits on involuntary hospitalizations.

The result is that thousands of mentally disabled persons have lost the protection of the state mental health systems and end up in unsavory locations, preyed upon by criminals, deteriorating physically, and often becoming the object of attention from the criminal justice system. In other words, if they become too obtrusive or disorderly, they land in jail, not a hospital.

Failure to take prescribed medication is a common problem with nonhospitalized mental patients, either because they dislike the side effects of the medicines or because they lack insight into the fact that they are ill.

A forty-year-old man with a long history of paranoid schizophrenia has the delusion that he is a government secret agent. He spends much of his time patrolling the city on various self-imposed "missions." Because of his conviction that he is not only well, but engaged in vital government work, he refuses to take the antipsychotic medications which have been recommended. During a recent nationwide attempt to eliminate "Social Security fraud," his disability benefits were discontinued. He contributed to this event by testifying convincingly that he was not disabled, but was, in fact, an employee of a government agency whose name he was not at liberty to reveal.

How the Health Care System Fosters Noncompliance

As Goffman (1961) has suggested, a patient's stay in the hospital would be much easier for the medical staff if the patient were not a person but, instead, a noninteracting object. When the medical plan does not take into account a patient's capacities, noncompliance is inevitable, as the following account illustrates. It resulted from a medical quest for the ideal medication regimen (ideal for managing the disease, not ideal from any other standpoint).

A. F., a widow in her late sixties, had multiple medical problems: a history of a stroke and two heart attacks as well as angina, hypertension, and diabetes. She felt she had nothing to live for except for her toy poodle, and she had become "overwhelmed" and unable to manage her own care. She was admitted to the hospital to stabilize her medically and to treat her suicidal depression. She responded well to psychotherapy, and discharge plans were made for Meals on Wheels and weekly contacts with a visiting nurse. Just before she was to be discharged, the patient was presented with the following medication schedule to which she was told she must strictly adhere if she were to avoid serious illness: Hydralazine, 4 times a day. (Omit if your systolic blood pressure is lower than 110). Quinidine, 4 times a day. Nifedipine, 3 times a day. (Omit if your systolic blood pressure is lower than 110). Potassium Chloride, 2 times a day. Furosemide, once a day in the morning. Metroprolol, 3 times a day. Isosorbide, every 6 hours. (Omit if your systolic blood pressure is lower than 110). Nitropaste. (Stagger this with the Isosorbide).

Faced with this proposal, the patient became agitated and begged to be kept in the hospital. She complained that she could not take her own blood pressure and that, even if she should learn to do it, she would be confined to home by this constant monitoring and would be unable to go to the store or to her church activities. She added that she was afraid of "poisoning" herself if she made a mistake in her medications. Hanson (see Chapter 9) discusses in depth the impact on compliance levels of such complex medical regimens.

The Medicalization of Social Problems

For some financially, socially, or psychologically disadvantaged patients, there are strong incentives for repeated hospitalizations. So long as the patient role inside the hospital or at the clinic is more attractive than the worker role in the community, patienthood can easily become addictive.

For those who have some chronic medical condition and who enjoy the sick role, noncompliance offers the ticket of admission. Examples are the diabetic in poor control because of dietary excesses, the cardiac patient who ignores risk factors, the alcoholic with exacerbation of gastrointestinal and liver problems, the paraplegic who "nurtures" a decubitus ulcer. Each of these examples of noncompliance (or indirect self-destructive behavior) can guarantee a hospital admission. As the following discussion indicates, Veterans Administration hospitals see many patients whose social problems are at least as pressing as their medical problems.

The Veterans Administration

The Veterans Administration system of health care, one of the largest in the world, was founded "to care for him who shall have borne the battle, and for his widow, and his orphan." Most persons unfamiliar with the VA assume that it treats only veterans who become wounded or ill during active service. This is not so. In fact, for the majority of the patients, the illness which brings them to a VA hospital is not service connected. Furthermore, the patients frequently suffer from financial and other social problems which the hospital staff tries to help solve. This active involvement of a medical institution in the nonmedical needs of its clients contributes to the long hospital stays for which the VA has been criticized. In 1982, the average length of stay for all VA medical centers was 14.8 days in contrast to 7.8 days for non-VA hospitals (VA Office of Reports and Statistics, 1983). The following account illustrates one of the reasons for this discrepancy in hospital stays.

> An otherwise healthy 60-year-old man has recovered uneventfully from gall bladder surgery, although he has been somewhat slow to get out of bed and says he still feels weak. On his 17th hospital day, he complains of increased pain in his finger, which has been stiff for 40 years as a result of a World War II shrapnel wound. An X-ray reveals no active disease process, and the physician proceeds to discharge the patient. The patient becomes enraged, shouts at the doctor, and strides off to consult his legal advisor at one of the veterans organizations.

The doctor is bewildered. What went wrong? The patient's behavior would seem rational if the doctor were aware that there is a rule that specifies that a service connected veteran who is treated for his service connected injury or illness during a hospitalization of at least 21 days receives a temporary increase in his Veterans Administration pension and is rated as 100% service connected. Thus, a person with a nominal residual impairment, such as a stiff finger, compensated at a 10% rate, can realize a substantial increase in his income if he can manage to spend 21 days in the hospital. At 1983 rates, the difference between 10% and 100% service connected disability is $1,151.00 per month.

The Role of Disability Compensation

The Workers Compensation system illustrates the adage that "every problem was once a solution." Conceived as a humane response to unprotected workers in an era when there was much arduous and dangerous work, it has become an increasing social burden. Ironically, as the work place has become safer, claims from injured workers have increased at an accelerating rate. This is also true of Social Security Disability awards. Between 1957 and 1976, these awards for low back pain increased by 2500 percent, more than five times the increase for lung cancer, which showed the next greatest increase (Social Security Administration, 1977–1979). Air traffic controllers have one of the highest rates of back injury claims, which shows that exposure to dangers on the job has little relation to the number of industrial injuries. In a study that demonstrated this fact, a careful evaluation was made of the movements required in certain jobs. As expected, workers rated "too weak" for their jobs had an excessive number of back injuries. However, this was also true of those who were rated "too strong" for their jobs (Loeser, 1983).

Society pays substantial costs for the increase in Workers Compensation claims. It has been estimated that 80% of the cost of each stamp we buy is used to pay for medical benefits and wage replacement for injured postal workers (Dicks, 1983).

Chronic low back pain is the most costly of the claims filed by injured workers. It is also one of the best examples of a problem which is more social, psychological, or financial than medical. It is generally accepted that soft tissue injuries to the low back should be healed in six months at the longest. When pain persists after that, it is usually treated with surgery, drugs, prolonged rest, or disability, all of which are very destructive to the well-being of the worker. The longer he is off work, the less likely he is to return to work, yet the system strings out his treatment until he is virtually unemployable (half of the workers with low back pain will never work again if they are off work more than 6 months).

Patients with chronic low back pain or other chronic nonmalignant pain typically fail to comply with treatment plans that require active and unpleasant effort on their part, such as weight loss or an exercise program. They prefer to take medicines and to refrain from most activities. They often engage in doctor shopping until they find a practitioner who advocates passive approaches like bed rest. This behavior pattern has been described as "killing with kindness" (Nehemkis & Cummings, 1982) and serves to perpetuate and even to increase both physical and mental impairment.

How Lawyers Thwart Compliance

The patient's lawyer is motivated to obtain the maximum financial recovery for the client, yet this means maximizing the associated pain and disability. These dual goals lead to the phenomenon of a patient entering a rehabilitation program, torn between his desire to feel better and the realization that if he shows significant improvement by complying with the treatment, his monetary award will be adversely affected.

Most patients are distressed enough to want the program to succeed. However, one sometimes realizes (unfortunately this is usually in retrospect) that a patient has entered a lengthy rehabilitation program with the covert goal of maintaining the state of disability so as to provide evidence in court of the intractability of his pain and disability.

More Paradoxes

We should like to draw attention to a second paradoxical situation in which health care providers find themselves at cross purposes. In an analysis of societally influenced chronic pain (Nehemkis & Cummings, 1982), we introduced the concept of "dysynchronous retirement." Dysynchronous retirement describes the sequence of events in which a laborer nearing the end of his working life sustains a relatively minor injury or flare-up of an old pain which becomes chronic and intractable. This condition legitimizes his status as a middle-aged retiree, out of synchrony with the retirement age prescribed by social custom.

There are very few old laborers or old construction workers. In one way or another, the system wears them out, and they have to tie an injury to the job in order to get medical care and compensation. This can lead to a "Catch-22" situation when periodic disability examinations are coupled with the expectation for compliance with the health care professionals who seek to reverse the chronicity of the very symptoms that free the patient from powerful social obligations.

In both instances described, one must note the inherent paradox or irony (a classic double bind from the patient's point of view) of demanding compliance to a regimen designed to alleviate or cure a disability which is a ticket to a larger lump sum settlement (in the case of the younger injured worker) or the continuation of a lifetime income (in the case of the dysynchronous retiree). The patient, the lawyer, the health care apparatus, and the private and public insurance systems of our society are absurdly pitted one against the other. The futility of attempting change, at the level of the individual patient and his physician, becomes obvious.

Restrictive Employment Criteria

Noncompliance with good health practices is reinforced when an injured worker is unable to get or keep work. Employers tend to overestimate vulnerability to reinjury with the attitude: "Once a bad back, always a bad back." The presence of a laminectomy scar on a job applicant's back will deter many employers from considering him further, although the job sought may involve no lifting or physical exertion. The prohibition extends even to those who have had back pain without surgery.

One of the nonmedical advantages of using Metrizamide rather than Pantopaque as a contrast medium for a myelogram is that it leaves no lasting trace. Pantopaque, which was the only medium available until recently, leaves a residue in the spinal canal which will show on x-rays in the future and signal to employers that this person once had a backache severe enough that surgery was contemplated.

Injured workers know that there are not jobs enough for all of them who have restrictions on sitting and standing. This is especially true of manual laborers who are considered too old for retraining. Why should they cooperate with a treatment regimen that will end with their being declared capable of working yet unable to get a job? Employers seldom welcome the injured worker back. Some heavy industries, like logging, produce more disabled persons than they can rehire. Injured workers are virtually one of the by-products of producing lumber, like sawdust or water pollution.

If employers do take back an injured worker, they are often unyielding when it comes to changing duties or work setting unless it is a physical necessity. This rigid approach is illustrated by the following examples:

A 35-year-old hospital worker was off work for a year and a half with a back injury and became heavily dependent on Valium and codeine. After six weeks in a pain management program, she was detoxified from these drugs and had become so physically fit that she wanted to return to work. She did not want to return to the storeroom where she had been injured because she had been unhappy with the supervisor and felt that the other workers thought she was malingering. Although she worked for a county government with thousands of employees and although she had clerical skills which could be used in other settings, the employer insisted that she return to her old work place. She missed work repeatedly because of recurring back pain, became angry and depressed, and finally accepted disability retirement.

A 30-year-old postal employee, with low back pain caused by an injury at work, was able to return to work after a long period of rehabilitation. His job required him to sit or lean on a sort of stool which increased his back pain. Despite his complaints and letters from two physicians, he was told that he could not be transferred to a more sedentary job or sit on a different stool and must continue to use this seat because it was approved by Occupational Safety and Health Act (OSHA) regulations. After several months, he ended up in the hospital having back surgery.

SENSE AND NONSENSE IN PATIENT COMPLIANCE

When is noncompliance rational? The early history of medicine is full of treatments which suggest that noncompliance might have been necessary for survival. When we read of the emetics, purges, and blood letting that helped speed George Washington through an upper respiratory infection and into the next world, we realize that "intelligent noncompliance" (Weintraub, 1976) could have saved many lives. As late as the turn of this century, mercury was recommended for the treatment of influenza and strychnine for the convalescent period (Davidson, 1982). Even in modern times, there have been many procedures that have been abandoned when they proved to be of no benefit. In regard to new drugs, there is a maxim that one should "use them fast, while they still work."

The consumer movement and the current emphasis on physical fitness are contemporary trends that bear on noncompliance. Both emphasize the responsibility of the individual to determine what is safe and healthy and to insist on having a say in the kind of medical care that is provided.

Sometimes this message is shrill, as on the cover of *Confessions of a Medical Heretic* (Mendelsohn, 1979), which warns "Caution: Medicine as practiced in America today may be dangerous to your health" and promises to tell "how to guard yourself against the harmful impact upon your life of doctors, drugs and hospitals." In the same vein, although with better documentation, is Illich's attack on the "medicalization of life" (1976). These books ask the consumer to view medicine with a critical eye, just like any other service. At best, this approach should encourage patients to ask appropriate questions and avoid overtreatment. At worst, it can lead to a paranoid view of the medical profession and a sort of therapeutic nihilism.

The same cautions apply to the physical fitness movement. Since so many chronic diseases are the product of unhealthy lifestyles, it is of obvious benefit if people are led to eat sensibly, stop smoking, drink less, and exercise regularly. Carried to an extreme, we have macrobiotic diets as the treatment of choice for cancer. A less eccentric example is the growing popularity of home births, sometimes with only a lay midwife in attendance. In a way, this is a tribute to the success of modern obstetrics, which is taken so much for granted that people do not realize that there could be any dangers connected with childbirth, once the major cause of death in young women.

Another contemporary site for noncompliance is the bedside of the terminally ill. In the era of antibiotics, pneumonia, "the old man's friend," no longer carries off those too ill or debilitated to want to live. The so-called "living will" is one response to the dilemma presented by prolonged, terminal, and painful illness. Measures that were once considered heroic are now part of routine intensive care. Physicians are realistically sensitive to the powerful legal sanctions against even the appearance of euthanasia. As a result, patients and their families must sometimes go to court for permission to refuse continued medical treatment or life-support systems for dying or hopelessly impaired patients.

We have given the least space to a discussion of poverty, certainly the most obvious social force for noncompliance. If they get sick enough, poor people will go to hospitals. However, short of extreme pain or life-threatening illness, they are forced to give a low priority to outpatient medical care. This is particularly true of preventive measures such as well-baby visits or dental checkups. Food and shelter come first.

THE ROLE OF THE CLINICIAN

Public health professionals are much concerned about citizens who smoke, refuse to use seat belts, skip immunizations and prenatal care, or fail to participate in other recommended routines and programs. Yet, as Udry and Morris (1971) point out, these measures are usually of much greater benefit to society as a whole than they are to any particular individual. For example, the risk of dying from lung cancer is significantly higher for smokers than for nonsmokers. However, this risk is still low enough (about one in a thousand per year for middle-aged male smokers) that a young smoker may not have a vivid sense of the mortality ratio in comparison to the immediate discomfort if he stops smoking.

A health cost that may not occur until much later in life is seen as a low cost when weighed against the bother or the costs in money or time that compliance would mean. In some low-risk diseases, the cost to society is great enough to justify unusual concessions to the consumer. This is the case with tuberculin testing which is provided free by health departments and is often made available at the work site as well. Where the social benefits are sufficiently great, preventive measures may be made compulsory, as in states that will not allow children to attend school without appropriate immunizations. It would appear that much noncompliance could be eliminated by enlarging the defined sphere of public interest so that preventive health care is made the responsibility of the government rather than left to indivudal discretion.

Short of legislating compliance, what can the clinician do when noncompliance is caused by societal forces? Patients are sometimes caught in a system that makes noncompliance seem the most reasonable choice. Labeling the patient as "uncooperative" or "resistant" is just a variation of "blaming the victim." Is it the patient's fault if the system of compensation makes it appear more rational to be noncompliant and disabled than to be compliant and ablebodied, but risk losing a job or an income? Our work places do not easily make a place for the injured worker. One result is what has been referred to as the career of the chronic pain patient. The blurring of the distinction between disability compensation and any other employment is nowhere shown more clearly than by a 32-year-old man with low back pain who stated that he would like to receive Social Security Disability because "I don't want my son to grow up on welfare."

Health care providers must become aware of the pressures on patients so that they do not take an unwitting role in an arrangement that is not therapeutic. For example, clinicians should not embark on a long, demanding, and expensive program of treatment if a patient's motivation is contaminated by legal advice or monetary self-interest. A physician can be most helpful by clarifying the issues to a patient in a supportive way.

It is also important to avoid getting into an adversary relationship with a noncompliant patient. Remember that noncompliance is not due to wickedness on the part of the patient. Malingering and self-inflicted injuries are rarely seen. One can only take a wry look at the societal forces that victimize patients and try to ally oneself with the patient's impulses toward health. The clinician can help the patient to realize that it is always better to be strong and healthy no matter what the incentives to maintain invalidism.

REFERENCES

Davidson, P. O. Issues in patient compliance. In T. Millan, C. Green, & R. Meagher (Eds.), *Handbook of clinical health psychology.* (pp. 417–434). New York: Plenum 1982.

Dicks, N. Our interdependency and responsibility in the problem of chronic back pain. In W. E. Fordyce (Chair), *Back pain, compensation and public policy.* Symposium conducted at the University of Washington, Seattle, May 1983.

Goffman, E. *Asylums.* Garden City, NY: Doubleday, 1961.

Illich, I. *Medical nemesis.* New York: Pantheon Books, 1976.

Loeser, J. D. An analysis of clinical pain. In W. E. Fordyce (Chair), *Back pain, compensation and public policy.* Symposium conducted at the University of Washington, Seattle, May 1983.

Mendelsohn, R. S. *Confessions of a medical heretic.* New York: Warner Books, 1979.

Nehemkis, A. M., & Cummings, C. The chronic pain syndrome: Killing with kindness. In M. G. Eisenberg, C. Griggins, & R. J. Duval (Eds.), *Disabled people as second-class citizens.* (pp. 217–231). New York: Springer, 1982.

Social Security Administration. *Social Security supplement 1977–1979.* (Table 129, p. 97; Table 130, p. 202).

Udry, J. R., & Morris, N. M. A spoonful of sugar helps the medicine go down. *American Journal of Public Health, 61,* 776–785, 1971.

Veterans Administration. *Summary of medical programs.* (p. 1). V.A. Office of Reports and Statistics, January 1983.

Weintraub, M. Intelligent noncompliance and capricious compliance. In L. Lasagna (Ed.), *Patient compliance.* Mt. Kisco, NY: Futura, 1976.

11

Epilogue:
The Complex Nature
of Compliance

Kenneth E. Gerber
Alexis M. Nehemkis

INTRODUCTION

The preceding chapters have presented a variety of perspectives from which to understand noncompliance in the chronically ill. We hope that the chapters will broaden the clinician's appreciation of the complexity of factors that determine noncompliant behavior. Chapter topics were chosen which would focus the reader's attention on aspects of noncompliance in chronic illness other than those most often addressed in the psychological treatment literature. The first part of this final chapter summarizes the alternative perspectives represented in this work while addressing treatment considerations suggested by a broadened understanding of noncompliance in the chronically ill. The chapter's second section suggests both general and specific areas for future clinical and research efforts.

Is Compliance Enough?

Davidson (1976), in addressing clinical problems associated with increasing compliance, develops a theme that supports the expanded conceptualization of compliance outlined in the present work. Davidson points out that the medical literature suggests that noncompliance is "vaguely sinful." Yet, the history of medicine demonstrates that perfect compliance with medical recommendation would often have been harmful to patients. Medical treatments, far from guaranteeing success, often have produced adverse effects on health. Furthermore, as Davidson suggests, identifying compliance as the ultimate value of medical intervention is a controversial proposition. We have observed that medical staff view their patients' compliance as a measure of their own professional success irrespective of how patients perceive the importance of complying to their own life satisfaction. Cohen and Lazarus (1979) remind us that the patient's taking less pain medication, complaining less, and complying perfectly with dietary restrictions reflects values related to the practical realities of the hospital/health care system. Only through the understanding of the patient's value system can we appreciate the meaning of the patient's response to recommendations and goals of the medical system. In the health care industry we continue to search for remedies that will provide a structure and rationale for compliance instead of capitulation to the relentless progression of chronic illness. In this book we have advanced the proposition that no single theoretical formulation or intervention strategy will be sufficient to solve all compliance problems, least of all those which arise (cf. Chapter 10) when a regimen is prescribed to alleviate or cure a disabling condition, the existence of which ensures the patient's continuing "financial health."

Regrettably, the compliance literature has for too long been cluttered with the results of the nomothetic approach—reams of data detailing the psychological, demographic, sociocultural, environmental, physiological correlates of compliant behavior. We share the view expressed by Kasl (1975) of much of the early compliance literature, in particular, as preoccupied with "superficial background variables" to the exclusion of fundamental theoretically derived attitudes and subjective perceptions. In her chapter on "Family Relationships and Compliance" Gervasio, in particular, makes a compelling case for the idiographic approach as a wellspring of information essential for understanding compliance.

In pondering that small number of factors with a confirmed relationship to noncompliance, some are decidedly more amenable to alteration than are others. Misconceptions and deeply ingrained stereotypic attitudes held by physicians and professional staff (Chapters 8 and 9) are *not* so easily changed. If and when, however, staff can recognize that the meaning of some episodes of noncompliance may be patients' attempts, for example, to solve an existential crisis (Chapter 5) or indirect self-destructive behavior that is, in the short run, "life-enhancing" (Chapter 3), this realization should, of its own accord, dictate the inappropriateness of many otherwise effective interventions. At the same time it should suggest the desirability of, for instance, a calculated posture of benign neglect, assumed by staff for the duration of the crisis, permitting the patient to work out his own destiny. At the very least, this realization on the part of the medical staff should enhance understanding and tolerance for the situation and perhaps thereby defuse any ill will that the noncompliance may have engendered. The discussion in Chapter 10 is particularly illuminating with respect to the kinds of noncompliant patterns that are impervious to change by virtue of our social welfare institutions and those which realistically may be subject to modification by the efforts of an individual clinician.

The Moral of A. F.

In Chapter 10 Cummings and Nehemkis introduced A.F., the widow in her late sixties, to illustrate a case of noncompliance made inevitable by the medical quest for the ideal medication regimen—ideal for managing the disease, not ideal from any other standpoint, as the authors duly note.

The case of A.F. provides a graphic illustration of the multidimensional barriers to compliance encountered by the geriatric patient and delineated by Amaral in Chapter 7: overprescription, intentional noncompliance in the face of polypharmacy, a regimen that doesn't consider the individual, and the presence of depressive symptomatology which can impede patient cooperation with any therapeutic regimen, even a simple one. Surely, A.F. would have fared better had a peer counselor and case coordinator been available to her to make follow-up calls, evaluate her progress, and assess her needs.

Theorists like Turk, Salovey, and Litt (Chapter 4) would

interpret A.F.'s panic and ensuing noncompliance as a predictable consequence of the failure to create a collaborative framework within which patient and health care provider work together to establish goals for self-care. "The health care provider must be willing to compromise and perhaps relinquish some components of an idealized regimen that will not be followed for one that may be less ideal but that has some likelihood of being followed" (p. 43).

Many of the contributors writing on the doctor–patient relationship, including, by inference, Hanson himself (Chapter 9), would view A.F.'s response as a form of iatrogenic noncompliance, that is, noncompliance which is initiated or exacerbated by the physician in one of a variety of ways. The early history of medicine is replete with examples suggesting that a patient's noncompliance was not infrequently a necessary precursor to survival. The example of A.F. should suggest that such cases cannot be dismissed as quaint curiosities and condescendingly consigned to the history book of prescientific medicine. While her pattern of admissions and chief complaints illustrate the medicalization of her loneliness and sense of betrayal, her difficulties with "doing what the doctor says" seem an appropriate response on the part of this elderly lady—an act of "intelligent noncompliance" to borrow Weintraub's (1976) term—to a pharmaceutical solution which does not take into account the human capacity to conform.

The Limits of Professional Responsibility

Several authors have raised the philosophical question of what therapeutic posture is to be adopted toward a patient's failure or repetitive failure to comply. Nehemkis and Gerber raise the issue in discussing "A Special Case of Noncompliance" (Chapter 5); namely, disengagement from the treatment relationship, where the failure to comply appears to be the patient's legitimate right. In Chapter 9, Hanson also addresses this issue: How far should a doctor go to make a patient appreciate that the cause of his obesity or the regulation of his hypertension is within his own control? He concludes that there are definable limits to the lengths that a physician need go, beyond the provision of information. Turk, Salovey, and Litt (Chapter 4), on the other hand, are

naturally inclined to view the failures to adhere as medical symptoms which necessitate a treatment regimen in the first place—that
is, as problems that can and should be solved. Their cognitive-
behavioral perspective dictates an approach in which they go to
elaborate and painstaking lengths, including even (1) the inculca-
tion of beliefs and values that are lacking and will have to be
instilled, such as the value of self-care in reducing long-term
complications and (2) the attempt to encourage patients to change
beliefs that may undermine compliance or help them come to
realize that their beliefs are maladaptive.

At the very least, the quest for meaningful compliance requires
that we acknowledge the disparity between what we, as health
care providers want and what can be expected in the not-too-
distant future. As Michael Weintraub observed in his notable
chapter entitled, 'Intelligent Noncompliance and Capricious
Compliance" (Weintraub, 1976):

> Current dogma holds that if treatment regimens are simplified with
> as few doses per day of the right color tablet, given with careful
> directions to patients conversant with the pathophysiology of their
> disease and the pharmacology of the drugs used in treating it, a
> state approaching therapeutic nirvana will be acheived. (p. 39)

Hence, we must not lose sight of the fact that effective compliance
does not always ensure cure, remission, or even good control of
the disease. Consider the prophetic observation of Achterberg-
Lawlis (1982):

> Behavioral compliance technology may represent an example of a
> technology having been developed in advance of an appropriate
> application in medicine. (p. 990)

When It Pays to Be Noncompliant

A good part of our failure to contain the problem of noncompliance is an outgrowth of our characteristic inclination to uni-
formly regard noncompliant behavior as something negative.
The reality is that noncompliance has both negative and positive
aspects. To appreciate this reality is to understand the layers of

positive meaning that noncompliant behavior may reflect. Indeed, there is a whole spectrum of payoffs for noncompliance, from the obvious to quite subtle, just as there is a whole range of patient motivations for such behavior, from the conscious and calculated to those only dimly perceived, if at all.

At one end of this positive spectrum of noncompliance will be found the many aspects of noncompliance that can be traced to the policies and programs of our modern industrial society: The Veterans Administration, SSI, Worker's Compensation, and restrictive employment criteria. These examples from Chapter 10 should make it apparent why some patients might choose the advantages of their disability over full compliance.

Somewhere in the middle of the spectrum of positive aspects lies noncompliance as hedonism. Here the behavior "pays" in terms of pleasurable gratification of rather immediate wants and needs or in the introduction of risk, excitement, and mastery into a life which otherwise feels dull and out of control (Chapter 3). At other times the payoff lies in the quest for renewed identity and self-validation, or in an act of protest against the medical fate which robs one of one's dreams. As Farberow puts it, "Many noncompliant acts are validational declarations of an inner core of self, indomitable and unconquered" (Chapter 3, p. 41).

Sometimes it is a matter of one's values, one's definition of quality of life, which determines when failure to comply with doctor's recommendations is rational or irrational. Thus, at the other end of the positive scale are those quality-of-life decisions best made by the patient, whose life it is after all. The reader will recall the advanced cancer patient, convinced of the truth of the adage that the treatment is worse than the disease, who elects to stop further chemotherapy (Chapter 5).

The preceding chapters have examined various facets of the positive side of noncompliance. Throughout, the authors have tried to convey how noncompliance at different times can work in opposite directions, so as both to impede or enhance the self and the patient's quality of life. But all too often debates in the literature at large ignore this underlying issue of the positive face of noncompliance and, as a result, the problem as a whole gets short shrift.

TREATMENT CONSIDERATIONS

Authors have addressed clinical issues in all of the preceding chapters. As the constant theme of this work has been to develop an appreciation of the complexity of noncompliant behavior, it is implicitly rejected that simplistic clinical strategies will effectively alter noncompliant behavior. We appreciate the utility of educational/informational interventions in certain cases in which patients valuing compliance with medical recommendations lack only specific direction or facts in order to achieve regimen adherence. We believe such cases to be few, particularly with the chronically ill who are constantly given information about their condition, yet still show high rates of nonadherence.

The efficacy of any psychotherapeutic intervention is best understood as relative. Patient characteristics, family dynamics, and staff idiosyncracies are all important, but none of these variables in and of itself is the critical sufficient condition determining optimal treatment response. Indeed, there is no one optimal treatment. No single psychological treatment is absolutely efficacious. They are all relative and must be judged only in the context of the meaning of the particular noncompliant behavior. Is it an indirect suicidal equivalent or a short-term self-enhancing coping strategy? Is it an attempt to alter or realign the power structure in the family as a result of the illness? Is it a response to and reflection of the psychosocial stage of the illness and accounted for by this more than any other cluster of variables? Is it the predictable response of a geriatric patient, subject to certain realities of old age, who has internalized society's negative stereotypes of old people and is behaving accordingly? Is it the patient's attempt to solve an existential crisis? Does the noncompliance have primary, or secondary, gain? Is it really not noncompliance at all, but behavior that disappoints or angers a staff whose expectations are unreasonable and whose attitudes are misconceived? Chapter 8, for instance, is not really about compliance as an objective truth, but rather about the way in which attitudes and perception shape what we call compliance. Different versions of noncompliance may be the products of perception and communication and not reflections of objective truths. Chapters

3, 6, 7, and 10 have implications for the type of interventions to apply once this evaluation has been made. Chapters 8 and 9 direct the reader's attention to the significant influence of patient-provider relationships on noncompliance and have implications for interventions involving staff attitude and expectations. Chapter 4 presents an integrated clinical assessment and treatment package expansive enough to accommodate both an empirically based approach with a concern for internal processes such as beliefs and values.

Treatment strategies for addressing noncompliance must reflect a thorough analysis of personal, social, and environmental factors which may influence patient behavior. None of the chapters was designed to offer specific treatment techniques such as those which reflect a behavioral technology. In that these methods are shortsighted and, in our experience, fail to increase appreciably regimen compliance in clinical populations, we could not recommend them as the preferred mode of treatment. The present work, by exploring a diversity of variables affecting the behavior of the chronically ill, will, we hope, lessen the distance yet to be covered in truly understanding the complex process of coping with chronic illness. As this understanding grows, effective treatment options will develop.

FUTURE DIRECTIONS

This volume has had as its major theme the notion that compliance is a complex, multidetermined phenomenon. Patients' compliance levels are the result of a myriad of influences, many of which we have addressed in this work. As Kaplan De-Nour succinctly states in the foreword, comprehensive research which analyzes the interaction of these separate factors is lacking. Without such analysis, interventions are difficult to design. Further, as the authors in this work have emphasized, the multiplicity of factors affecting compliance level reinforces the necessity of individualizing treatment as each case is, ultimately, unique and complex. Another general recommendation for future effort is also mentioned in Kaplan De-Nour's Foreword to this volume. The dearth of physician involvement in the greater understanding of compliance is a clear shortcoming. The medical recommendations patients are expected to comply with, after all, are most often directed from physicians. The development of greater sensitivity of physicians, particularly those in training, to the underlying issues affecting compliance should represent a major effort of future research and medical education.

All of the chapters in this book suggest numerous directions for future research and clinical efforts. The complex determinants of how patients become labeled as noncompliant, we believe, are an important area for future research. Further delineation, through multifactorial technique, of how social psychological variables affect the labeling process could provide valuable insight into how factors irrelevant to actual patient behavior determine, often falsely, how patients are viewed by others. We have seen, for example, that patients are labeled as noncompliant for a myriad of reasons (e.g., likability, similarity to caregivers) unrelated to the actual degree of compliance with medical regimen. Another area in major need of further research investigation is that of the family impact on coping with chronic illness. As Gervasio emphasizes (Chapter 6), the family role in influencing patient compliance has not been made clear in previous research. It is not well understood which type of intervention into the family system would most effectively enhance patient compliance. Related to the issue of family influence is greater investigation into the unique factors affecting that segment of the population most vulnerable to chronic disease—the elderly. The delineation of how the many significant variables, environmental, social, economic, cognitive, and emotional influence compliance levels has not, as Amaral states, been effectively addressed in the research literature. Comprehensive intervention programs attentive to the myriad of even seemingly minor factors such as transportation or institutional design would seem to ensure more effective adherence to necessary medical recommendations. More generally, Turk, Salovey, and Litt encourage the development of innovative approaches to increase patients' sense of responsibility for and perceived competence in effectively coping with their illness.

In keeping with the cognitive-behavioral focus, future emphasis should be on the development of treatment methods compatible with the interactive view of this model.

Finally, in keeping with a major focus of this book, we believe that the greater understanding of compliance must include an appreciation of certain moral questions. Although such questions are, inevitably, unanswerable, their consideration is necessary in order to achieve the broadened perspective on compliance which this book has repeatedly stressed. Zaner (1981), a philosopher, has addressed these matters in reference to hemodialysis patients, but this discussion is relevant to all individuals with chronic disease. He reminds us that the judgment of a patient's desire to life, cooperativeness, or emotional stability reflects the values of the outsider and are, ultimately, ethical matters. The dilemma of the chronically ill individual, then, is most fundamentally a moral one, nothing less than the complex determination of how individuals should live given their unique life circumstances.

REFERENCES

Achterberg-Lawlis, J. The psychological dimensions of arthritis. *Journal of Consulting and Clinical Psychology, 50*(6), 984–992, 1982.

Cohen, F., & Lazarus, R. S. Coping with the stresses of illness. In G. C. Stone, F. Cohen, & N. E. Adler (Eds.), *Health psychology.* San Francisco: Jossey-Bass, 1979.

Davidson, P. Therapeutic compliance. *Canadian Psychological Review, 17,* 247–259, 1976.

Holroyd, K. A., & Lazarus, R. S. Stress, coping and somatic adaptation. In L. Goldberger & S. Breznitz (Eds.), *Handbook of stress: theoretical and clinical aspects.* New York: Free Press, 1982.

Kasl, S. V. Issues in patient adherence to health care regimens. *Journal of Human Stress, 1,* 5–17, 1975.

Weintraub, M. Intelligent noncompliance and capricious compliance. In L. Lasagna (Ed.), *Patient compliance.* Mt. Kisco, NY: Futura, 1976.

Zaner, R. Dialysis and ethics: Be strong and trust (please!) In B. Levy (Ed.), *PsychoNephrology I,* New York: Plenum, 1981.

Zifferblatt, S. M. Increasing patient compliance through the applied analysis of behavior. *Preventive Medicine, 4,* 173–182, 1975.

Index

Adherence
  cognitive-behavioral enhancement
    of, 53–67
  cognitive-behavioral perspective
    on, 44–69
  vs. compliance, 12–13, 44–45;
    see also Compliance
  phases of, 68 (tab.)
Age, ISDB and, 38
Alcohol abuse
  and noncompliant ISDB, 37
  relapse prevention, 66

Behavioral theories of families, 106–
  108
Beliefs, patient, and adherence, 49
Buerger's disease, 30–32

Cancer
  compliance with treatment, 90–
    95
  among the elderly, 130
  perceptions of life changes from,
    162–163
  staff attitudes toward, 165–167
  terminal stage and noncompliance,
    94–95
Center for the Partially Sighted,
  151–153
Chemotherapy, see Cancer
Chronic illness
  and compliance, overview of, 12–
    21
  in elderly, see Elderly chronically
    ill
  overview of problems, 1–5
Cognitive-behavioral approach to ad-
    herence (compliance), 7, 44–
    69, 87–88
  cognitive restructuring, 59–60
  collaborative framework, 53–54
  contingency contracting, 60–63
  enhancing adherence, 53–67

intervention strategies, 17–18
model, 46–52
phases of adherence, 68 (tab.)
problem-solving approach, 54–58
provision of information, 58–59
relapse prevention, 64–67
restructuring staff attitudes and
  expectations, 174–175
social support, 63–64
stress inoculation, 64–67
Cognitive-behavioral model of ad-
    herence to self-care regimens,
    46–52
  action, 51
  beliefs, 49
  feedback, 52
  knowledge and skills, 47–49
  motivation, 50–51
Cognitive restructuring, 59–60
Collaborative framework in enhanc-
    ing adherence, 53–54
Compliance
  adaptive, 40
  vs. adherence, 12–13, 44–45; see
    also Adherence
  complex nature of, 226–235
  vs. conformity, 39–40
  definition of, 12–13
  extent of need for, 176–178
  factors affecting, 15–16
  future research directions on,
    233–235
  intervention strategies to increase,
    16–18
  limits of, 203–207
  limits of professional responsibil-
    ity, 229–230
  negative aspects of, 39–40
  overview of, 12–21
  phases of, 68 (tab.)
  positive aspects of, 40
  see also Noncompliance
Compliance specialists, 202–203
Conformity, compliance and, 39–40

Consumer movement, noncompliance and, 222
Contingency contracting, 60–63
Continuous ambulatory peritoneal dialysis (CAPD), 76–77; *see also* Dialysis
Coping, noncompliance and, 18–21
Cults, compliance and, 40

Demographic variables
  and compliance, 15
  and family support, 99–100
Denial, *see* Self-destructive behavior, indirect
Dependency, patient, covert demands for, 171–172
Diabetes, 14, 15
  among the elderly, 129–130
  and noncompliant ISDB, 28–30
  patient's knowledge of, and adherence, 47–48
Dialysis
  behavioral approach to noncompliance, 87–88
  and compliance, 2–5, 8, 19, 77–78, 85–86
  continuous ambulatory peritoneal, 76–77
  evolution and history of, 74–75
  existential dilemma in, 79–80
  intervention program to counter staff bias in, 173–174
  noncompliance as solution to existential crisis, 88–90
  and noncompliant ISDB, 34–35
  patient compliance as staff problem, 80–84
  physical complications of, 75–76
  problems of patients in, 74–77
  quality of survival in, 73–90
  staff vs. patient perceptions of life changes in, 160
  "too long life" problem, 78–79
Disability compensation, 218–219
Drug abuse, 26, 27
  treatment programs and noncompliant ISDB, 35–39
Dysynchronous retirement, 219–220

Elderly chronically ill, 9–10, 128–154
  Center for Partially Sighted program, 151–153
  and cognitive impairment, 143–144
  compliance patterns, 131–132
  and depression, 144–145
  enhancing compliance, 147–153
  environmental barriers to compliance, 135–143
  health problems, range of, 129–132
  and hearing problems, 134–135
  inadequate therapeutic regimens for, 137–143
  and income problems, 135–136
  multiplicity of problems as barrier to compliance, 146–147
  and noncompliant ISDB, 32–33
  over-prescription for, 137–140
  physical barriers to compliance, 133–135
  psychological barriers to compliance, 143–146
  and self-image, 145–146
  and social isolation problems, 136–137
  and transportation problems, 136
  and visual problems, 133–134
Existential crisis in chronic illness, 79–80, 88–90
Expectations, incongruent, and noncompliance, 167–169

Family functioning, theories of, 105–113
  behavioral, 106–109
  family systems, 109–113
  psychoanalytic, 106
Family relations and compliance, 7–8, 98–124
  case studies, 113–123
  enmeshment and communication patterns, 121–123
  homeostasis and role changes, 114–117
  intervention, 123–124
  research on, 99–105
  theories of family functioning, 105–113
  triangulation, 117–121
Family roles, research on, 100–102
Family support, research on, 102–103
Family systems theory, 109–113
Feedback, adherence and, 52

Health care team, *see* Physician-

patient relationship; Staff
perceptions of noncompliance
Hemodialysis, *see* Dialysis
Hyperobesity
and noncompliant ISDB, 33–34
self-care programs, family support
and, 64
Hypertension, 14–15, 129

Indirect self-destructive behavior
(ISDB), *see* Self-destructive
behavior, indirect
Information provision to patient, 47–
49, 58–59, 183–184

Knowledge, patient, and adherence,
47–49

Lawyers, patient's, and noncompliance, 219
Low back pain, chronic, 6, 218–219

Mental patients, nonhospitalized, noncompliance among, 214–215
Methadone maintenance program,
noncompliant ISDB and, 35–39
Motivation, patient, and adherence,
50–51
Mutual participation model of physician-patient relationship, 193–
196

Noncompliance
in cancer treatment, 93–94
cognitive-behavioral approach to,
87–88; *see also* Cognitive behavioral approach to adherence
and coping process, 18–21
in dialysis treatment, *see* Dialysis
extent of, 13–15
and family relationships, *see* Family relations and compliance
iatrogenic, 228–229
limits of professional responsibility, 229–230
positive aspects of, 230–231
as solution to existential crisis, 88–
90
staff perceptions of, *see* Staff perceptions of noncompliance
treatment considerations, 232–233
see also Adherence; Compliance

Noncompliance specialists, 202–203
Nurse-patient relationship, *see* Staff
perceptions of noncompliance

Obesity, *see* Hyperobesity
Oncology, *see* Cancer
Osteoarthritis, 130

Pain, staff attitudes toward patient,
163–165
Patient perceptions
and compliance, 16
vs. staff perceptions of life changes
in chronic illness, 159–163
Physical fitness movement, noncompliance and, 222–223
Physician-patient relationship, 8,
182–208
assessing compliance, 190–191
assessing reasons for noncompliance, 191–193
communication of information,
183–184
interactional variables, 187–189
limits of compliance, 203–207
limits of professional responsibility in noncompliance, 229–230
models of, 193–197
patient variables, 186–187
physician variables, 184–186
physician's influence on patient
compliance, 189–203
social influence and social power,
role of, 197–201
and societal contributions to noncompliance, 223–225
see also Staff perceptions of noncompliance
Physician-patient relationship models,
193–196
Power, social, 197–201
Problem-solving approach to self-care
regimens, 54–58
Psychiatric treatment programs
and noncompliant ISDB, 35–38
nonhospitalized patients, 214–215
Psychoanalytic theory of families, 106

Quality of life, compliance and, 17–
18, 73–95
cancer, 73, 90–95
chronic hemodialysis, 73–90

Referred power, 200–201
Reinforcement, adherence and, 50–51
Relapse prevention in self-care prog-
    rams, 64–67
Renal failure, *see* Dialysis
Restrictive employment criteria, non-
    compliance and, 220–221
Risk-taking, 27, 28, 41; *see also*
    Self-destructive behavior, in-
    direct
Role reversal in self-care, training, 58–
    59

Self-abuse, *see* Self-destructive behav-
    ior, indirect
Self-care programs
    cognitive-behavioral model in,
        46–52
    enhancing adherence to, 53–67
Self-destructive behavior, indirect
    (ISDB), 9, 24–41
    and Buerger's disease, 30–32
    case file study, 35–39
    clinical aspects of, 39–41
    definition of, 25–28
    in delinquency treatment prog-
        rams, 35–39
    and diabetes, 28–30
    and dialysis, 34–35
    in drug treatment programs, 35–39
    and elderly chronically ill, 32–33
    and hyperobesity, 33–34
    and psychiatric treatment prog-
        rams, 35–39
Self-report measures, patient, 15
Skills, patient, and adherence, 47–49
Smoking, 14, 30–32
Social power, 197–201
Social support in self-care programs,
    63–64
Societal contributions to noncompli-
    ance, 5–6, 213–225
    disability compensation, 218–219
    dysynchronous retirement, 219–
        220
    factors impeding treatment of
        chronically ill, 214–215
    health care system's role in non-
        compliance, 215-216
    lawyers, patient's, and, 219
    medicalization of social problems,
        216-217

and physician-patient relationship,
    197–201
    restrictive employment criteria,
        220–221
    role of clinician, 223–225
    sense and nonsense in patient com-
        pliance, 222–223
    Veterans Administration, 217–218
Staff perceptions of noncompliance,
    8, 158–178
    cognitive-behavioral approach in re-
        structuring staff attitudes and
        expectations, 174–175
    and covert demands for patient de-
        pendency, 171–172
    designing an intervention program
        to counter staff bias, 172–174
    determinants of, 169–171
    in dialysis treatment, 80–84
    extent of need for compliance,
        176–178
    noncompliance due to incongruent
        expectations, 167–169
    in oncology unit, 165–167
    pain, importance of, 163–165
    vs. patient perceptions of life
        changes in chronic illness, 159–
        163
    role of staff in compliance, 201–
        203
    team treatment concept, reserva-
        tions on, 175–176
Stress inoculation in self-care prog-
    rams, 64–67
Structural family therapy, 111–112
Suicide, noncompliant ISDB and, 36–
    38

Terminal illness, noncompliance and,
    94–95, 223
Thromboangiitis obliterans (Buerger's
    disease), 30–32

Value changes of chronically ill, 161–
    163
Veterans Administration, 217–218

Workers Compensation, 218–219

Youth delinquency programs, non-
    compliant ISDB and, 35–39